Antiviral Chemotherapy, Interferons and Vaccines

Monographs in Virology

Vol. 16

Editor: *J. L. Melnick,* Houston, Tex.

KARGER

S. Karger · Basel · München · Paris · London · New York · Tokyo · Sydney

Antiviral Chemotherapy, Interferons and Vaccines

David O. White

Department of Microbiology, University of Melbourne,
Parkville, Vic., Australia

5 figures and 13 tables, 1984

KARGER

S. Karger · Basel · München · Paris · London · New York · Tokyo · Sydney

Monographs in Virology

National Library of Medicine, Cataloging in Publication
White, David O.
Antiviral Chemotherapy, interferons and vaccines
David O. White, – Basel; New York: Karger, 1984. –
(Monographs in virology; v. 16)
Includes index.
1. Antiviral Agents – therapeutic use 2. Interferons 3. Viral Vaccines 4. Virus Diseases – drug therapy 5. Virus Diseases – prevention & control I. Title II. Series
W1 MO569P v. 16 [QV 268.5 W583a]
ISBN 3-8055-3825-1

Drug Dosage

The authors and the publisher have exerted every effort to ensure that drug selection and dosage set forth in this text are in accord with current recommendations and practice at the time of publication. However, in view of ongoing research, changes in government regulations, and the constant flow of information relating to drug therapy and drug reactions, the reader is urged to check the package insert for each drug for any change in indications and dosage and for added warnings and precautions. This is particularly important when the recommended agent is a new and/or infrequently employed drug.

Printed in Switzerland by Reinhardt AG, Basel
ISBN 3-8055-3825-1

Contents

Antiviral Chemotherapy

I. Introduction

The fact that the replication of all viruses is absolutely dependent upon essential metabolic pathways of the host cell presents a greater challenge to those seeking antiviral chemotherapeutic agents than faced the pioneers of antibacterial chemotherapy. Not surprisingly therefore, progress has been slow since the discovery of the naturally occurring antiviral agent interferon in 1956 so clearly demonstrated the feasibility of antiviral chemotherapy. The search has been largely empirical, many of the agents described so far having been discovered during random or serendipitous screening of naturally occurring, e.g. fungal, substances for anticancer activity [*Shannon and Schabel,* 1980; *de Clercq,* 1981]. Furthermore, the cost of developing a new chemotherapeutic agent has increased enormously since governmental regulatory agencies such as the Food and Drug Administration in the United States, alarmed by the thalidomide disaster, began in 1962 to demand far more comprehensive evidence of lack of teratogenicity and carcinogenicity as well as toxigenicity in man. *Grunert* [1979] estimated that the minimum delay between discovery of a new drug and its licensing for human administration had extended to 8 years, and the development cost to at least $ 50 million (in 1976 dollars!). Partly for this reason, pharmaceutical companies have concentrated their efforts on a search for agents against the more prevalent human viruses, and viruses of economic importance in animals. By and large, the harvest from their investment has been rather disappointing.

II. Strategy for Development of Antiviral Agents

In recent years our deepening understanding of the molecular biology of viral replication has led to a more rational approach to the search for antiviral chemotherapeutic agents. We now recognize a considerable number of steps in the viral multiplication cycle which represent potential targets for selective attack. In particular, all virus-coded enzymes are theoretically vulnerable, as are all processes (enzymatic or nonenzymatic) that are more essential to the multiplication of the virus than to the survival of the cell. Obvious examples include (1) transcription of viral mRNA (or cDNA, in the case of the retroviruses) by the viral transcriptase; (2) replication of viral DNA or RNA by the virus-coded DNA polymerase or RNA-dependent RNA polymerase; (3) post-translational cleavage of protein(s) by (virus-coded) protease(s). Less obvious at first sight, but proven points of action of currently known antiviral agents are: (4) entry/uncoating; (5) polyadenylation, methylation or capping of viral mRNA; (6) translation of viral mRNA into protein; and (7) assembly/maturation of the virion [*Becker and Hadar,* 1980; *Elion,* 1980; *Smith* et al., 1980; *Becker,* 1982; *de Clercq,* 1982a, c].

The recent discovery of a new class of nucleoside analogues which selectively inhibit herpesvirus DNA synthesis has opened our eyes to the fact that virus-coded enzymes with a broader (or simply different) substrate specificity than their cellular counterparts can be exploited to convert an inactive 'precursor' drug to an active antiviral agent. Because the viral enzyme occurs only in infected cells, such drugs are nontoxic for uninfected cells [*Elion,* 1980; *de Clercq,* 1981, 1982a, c]. Exploitation of this principle may revolutionize antiviral chemotherapy.

A logical approach to the discovery of new antiviral chemotherapeutic agents is to isolate or synthesize substances that might be predicted to serve as a substrate or inhibitor of a known virus-coded enzyme. Having found an agent which, in its native state or following modification by a virus-coded enzyme, displays a degree of specificity for a viral enzyme, synthetic pathway or any other process integral to the viral replication

Table I. Animal models for testing antiviral agents

Virus	Animal	Route
Herpes simplex 1	rabbit	ocular
	rabbit, guinea pig, mouse	dermal
Herpes simplex 2	guinea pig	genital
Varicella-zoster[a]	patas monkey	parenteral
Cytomegalovirus[a]	mouse	parenteral
Influenza	ferret, mouse, squirrel monkey	intranasal
Rhinovirus	chimpanzee, gibbon, man	intranasal
Respiratory syncytial	hamster, ferret, cotton rat, chimpanzee	intranasal
Rotavirus[a]	piglet, calf, mouse, tree-shrew	oral
Calicivirus[a]	cat, piglet	oral
Enterovirus[a]	mouse	oral
Hepatitis A	marmoset	oral
Hepatitis B	chimpanzee	parenteral
Togavirus	mouse	parenteral, intracerebral

[a] In these cases the human virus does not multiply satisfactorily, hence model viruses of the same genus which are native to the laboratory hosts listed are used.

cycle, analogues (congeners) of this prototype are now synthesized with a view to enhancing activity and/or selectivity. Inhibition of activity of a particular viral enzyme, e.g. DNA polymerase or reverse transcriptase, may be assayed directly in vitro, and techniques such as cryoenzymology, X-ray crystallography and nuclear magnetic resonance harnessed to elucidate structural imperatives. Recombinant DNA technology should facilitate and expedite the search, because it should soon be almost a matter of routine to clone any viral gene, sequence it and/or its protein product, purify and crystallize the protein, solve its tertiary structure by X-ray crystallography, identify its active site(s), and design competitive inhibitors.

Ultimately, however, the critical test of any putative chemotherapeutic agent must be inhibition of viral multiplication. Suitable indicator viruses, such as herpes simplex, influenza, rhinoviruses, etc., are assayed for plaque reduction in dilutions of the agent. Toxicity of the drug for human cells may be measured crudely by cytopathic effect (CPE) (in the absence of virus) or, more sensitively, by reduction in plating efficiency or cell-doubling time. The 'therapeutic index' may be defined as the ratio of the minimum cell-toxic dose to minimum virus-inhibitory dose. In general, only those agents displaying a therapeutic index of at least ten and preferably 100–1,000 are worth pursuing further. The literature is cluttered with worthless reports of 'antiviral' agents that are lethal for cells. Indeed, many agents that look promising in cell culture also fall by the wayside at the next hurdle, namely the experimental animal. Some typical test systems are listed in table I. Of course, for some human viruses no suitable animal model exists; potential chemotherapeutic agents against common cold viruses, for example, have often been assayed first in organ culture, then directly in human volunteers.

Before embarking on clinical trials in man, the pharmacology and toxicology of the drug must be thoroughly investigated in experimental animals, including, desirably, primates. Ideally, the drug should be water-soluble, chemically and metabolically stable, and moderately apolar, and it must be taken into cells. Pharmacokinetic studies address such questions as the mechanism and rate of absorption following various routes of administration, tissue distribution, metabolism (detoxification) and excretion of the drug. Tests for acute toxicity encompass comprehensive clinical surveillance of all the body systems, biochemical tests (e.g. for liver and kidney function), hematological examination, tests for immunosuppression, and so on. Longer-term investigations screen for chronic toxicity, allergenicity, mutagenicity, carcinogenicity, and teratogenicity [reviews: *Herrmann,* 1977; *Oxford,* 1977; *Grunert,* 1979].

III. Clinical Application of Antiviral Chemotherapy

A. Route of Administration

The route of administration of an antiviral agent is a prime consideration in assessing its general acceptability. The oral route is naturally much the most convenient for the patient, and perhaps the only one he will tolerate for the treatment of trivial disease. Nasal drops or sprays may be acceptable for upper respiratory infections but can be irritating. Topical preparations are also satisfactory for localized superficial infections of skin or eye, but not for generalized skin or genital infections. Parenteral administration, though unpopular with patients, may be required for serious systemic infections. Intravenous infusion of course necessitates hospitalization. In veterinary medicine, injection is generally the optimum route of delivery.

Some novel mechanisms of delivery of antiviral drugs have recently been suggested. *Knight* et al. [1980, 1981] have delivered ribavirin and amantadine to influenza patients by inhalation (for up to 60 h through a face mask) of a small-particle aerosol generated by a nebulizer. The blood-brain barrier, which constitutes an impediment to the treatment of encephalitis by some drugs, can be reversibly breached, in rats at least, by infusing a hyperosmotic solution of arabinose into the external carotid artery [*Barranger* et al., 1979]. It has been postulated that antiviral drugs applied to recurrent herpetic skin lesions might be selectively delivered to sites of latent infection in ganglia by coupling them to substances known to undergo retrograde axonal transport [*Fox and White,* 1980]. Various procedures have been tried to enhance the penetration of antiviral drugs into the skin: whereas dimethyl sulfoxide [*Juel-Jensen,* 1970] has not been licensed for general use, polyethylene glycol [*Spruance* et al., 1982] may turn out to be almost as effective; iontophoresis [*Hill* et al., 1977] has been claimed to increase the effectiveness of antiviral agents in genital herpes; local hyperthermia has been employed to facilitate release of drugs from liposomes [*Yatvin* et al., 1978]. Indeed, *Gregoriadis* [1976] has advocated the more general use of multilamellar liposomes for systemic delivery of antiviral agents to other sites in the body. However, since most are wasted as a result of being taken up by phagocytic cells, in local lymph nodes following intramuscular injection, or liver and spleen following intravenous inoculation, he made the further suggestion that such drug-containing liposomes might be coated with antiviral antibody to direct them to infected target cells [*Gregoriadis,* 1980]. Direct conjugation of antiviral agents to antibodies recognizing viral antigens on infected cells is also an approach worth exploring, as is currently being done for anticancer therapy [*Möller,* 1982a].

B. Drug-Resistant Mutants

It is already clear that mutants resistant to many of the available antiviral drugs readily emerge in vitro and in vivo. These inevitable occurrences will have to be faced in much the same way as we have learned to live with the problem of antibiotic-resistant bacteria. Antiviral agents will need to be used only when absolutely necessary, but then applied in adequate dosage. Certain life-saving drugs may need to be retained for designated diseases only. Combined therapy, using agents with distinct modes of action, would be expected to reduce the probability of selection of resistant mutants – as well as to minimize potential toxic side effects and, in certain instances, to display synergism, as has been claimed for interferon + adenine arabinoside monophosphate (ara-AMP), interferon + acyclovir, adenine arabinoside (ara-A) + acyclovir, and ribavirin + amantadine, for example. Mutants would not be expected to arise nearly as readily against drugs with multiple points of action – interferons are an obvious case in point, but the same may be true for other present and future antiviral agents, e.g., ara-A and ribavirin.

C. Clinical Priorities

Diseases with a large number of different etiological agents are prime targets for antiviral chemotherapy, as are those against which no satisfactory vaccine is available; the common cold is an admirable example on both counts. Other upper respiratory infections, gastroenteritis, hepatitis and infectious mononucleosis, must also be high on the list of priorities. Recurrent episodes of herpes simplex and zoster are singularly troublesome, and effective chemotherapy would be a boon, although the latent infection itself is unlikely to be eradicated. Chronic and slow virus infections may be particularly amenable to antiviral chemotherapy, as might some other long drawn out diseases of currently unknown etiology such as certain cancers, autoimmune diseases and degenerative conditions of the brain, should any of these, in the fullness of time, turn out to be of viral causation. Finally, we must not neglect the rarer, lethal viral diseases, such as rabies, poliomyelitis, encephalitis and the hemorrhagic fevers, for which successful chemotherapy would be life-saving.

Acute infections may need to be treated promptly, at the time of appearance of the first prodromal symptom, e.g., the 'tingling' (paresthesia) of recurrent herpes simplex or zoster, or the nasal congestion of the common cold or the exanthemata. Relatively broad-spectrum chemotherapeutic agents will be needed if treatment is to be commenced before a definitive diagnosis has been established. Otherwise, rapid diagnostic techniques such as ELISA (EIA), immunofluorescence, or IgM serology will be essential to select the appropriate drug for treatment.

Chemoprophylaxis may also have a role, not only in the prevention of complications such as orchitis or meningitis in mumps, but also in protection against the spread of diseases like hepatitis, mononucleosis, polio, influenza, measles or rubella to unimmunized family contacts.

D. Antibacterial Chemotherapy

Finally, it is relevant to comment on the use of antibacterial agents in the treatment of viral diseases. Physicians the world over tend to overprescribe antibiotics, not only for unspecified infections, but even for viral infections against which they (should) know conventional antibiotics are totally impotent. Such irresponsible medicine should be strongly discouraged. The only circumstances justifying the use of antibacterial antibiotics in the treatment of viral infections are the following: (1) to 'play safe' pending the laboratory identification of the etiological agent in the case of serious illnesses where there is real diagnostic doubt about the possibility of a bacterial cause, e.g., meningitis or pneumonia; and (2) to prevent serious bacterial superinfection of a viral disease, e.g., the secondary development of otitis media or pneumonia in a bronchiectatic child with measles, or bronchopneumonia in an elderly cardiac or pulmonary invalid with influenza.

Following two decades of rather disappointing progress, we have witnessed something of a resurgence in the field of antiviral chemotherapy since the late 1970s. Interferons and the 'second-generation' nucleoside derivatives look particularly promising. These and other selected agents will be discussed in a certain amount of detail below. To attempt a comprehensive survey of all the compounds reported in the literature to display promise in vitro would be foolhardy and misleading. Even some of those claimed to show selectivity in man have been omitted so that we might concentrate on those that seem at the time of writing (late 1982) to be of real potential value or to illustrate important principles or new directions. Readers seeking more comprehensive listings are referred to the following large selection of recent books and reviews: *Bauer* [1977, 1980a], *Becker* [1976, 1982], *Becker and Hadar* [1980], *Came and Caliguiri* [1982], *Collier and Oxford* [1980], *Couch and Jackson* [1976], *de Clercq* [1979, 1981, 1982a, c], *Elion* [1980], *Galasso* [1981a, b], *Galasso* et al. [1979], *Hahn* [1980], *Herrmann* [1977], *Hirsch and Swartz* [1980], *Merigan* [1976, 1981a, b], *Oxford* [1977], *Richman and Oxman* [1978], *Shannon and Schabel* 1980], *Smith* et al. [1980], *Swallow* [1978], *Walker* et al. [1979], *Whitley and Alford* [1978, 1981].

IV. Interferons

A. Overview

More than a quarter of a century has passed since *Isaacs and Lindenmann* [1957] described a protein, 'interferon', which is produced by virus-infected cells and protects uninfected cells against viral infection. Ever since, it has been evident that interferon is, in theory at least, the ideal antiviral antibiotic. It is naturally occurring, relatively nontoxic, and displays a broad spectrum of activity against essentially all viruses [for comprehensive reviews see the following recent books: *Baron* et al., 1982; *Came and Carter,* 1983; *de Maeyer and Schellekens,* 1983; *de Maeyer* et al., 1981; *Finter* et al., 1984; *Friedman,* 1981; *Gresser,* 1979, 1980, 1981, 1982; *Kono,* 1982; *Merigan and Friedman,* 1982; *Pestka,* 1981; *Stewart,* 1979; *Stringfellow,* 1980a; *Vilček* et al., 1980]. Yet, clinical trials in man had been generally disappointing until techniques for the purification of human interferon were developed in the late 1970s and opened the way for trials which demonstrated that interferon at much higher dosage could be effective against at least some viral diseases [reviews: *Dunnick and Galasso,* 1979, 1980; *Merigan,* 1981a, b; *Came and Carter,* 1983; *Kono,* 1982; *Munk and Kirchner,* 1982; *World Health Organization,* 1982] and perhaps even against some cancers [reviews: *Gresser and Tovey,* 1978; *Dunnick and Galasso,* 1979, 1980; *de Maeyer* et al., 1981; *Merigan,* 1981a, b; *Baron* et al., 1982; *Munk and Kirchner,* 1982; *Pollard,* 1982].

The recent cloning of the genes for human interferons in bacteria [*Nagata* et al., 1980; *Goeddel* et al., 1980b; *Derynck* et al., 1980; *Taniguchi* et al., 1980a, b], then in yeasts [*Hitzeman* et al., 1981], and finally in mammalian cells [*Gray* et al., 1982; *Mantei and Weissmann,* 1982] represents one of the great triumphs of recombinant DNA technology. Not only has this breakthrough greatly reduced the cost of interferon but it has led to the realization that there are in fact many separate human genes, situated mainly on chromosomes 9 [*Burke and Meager,* 1980; *Owerbach* et al., 1981; *Sehgal* et al., 1981] and 12 [*Naylor* et al., 1983], coding for at

Table II. Physicochemical properties of human interferons

Property	α	β	γ
Previous designations	Le–IFN type I	F–IFN type I	immune IFN type II
Subtypes	>12	1 (? more)	1 (?2)
Mr			
Major subtypes	15,000–25,000	20,000	20,000–25,000
Cloned (non-glycosylated)	19,000	19,600	17,110
Glycosylation	no[a]	yes	yes
pH 2 stability	stable[a]	stable	labile
Induction	viruses	viruses	mitogens
Principal source	lymphocyte, etc.	fibroblast	lymphocyte
Activity in bovine cells	yes	no	no
Introns in gene	no	no	yes
Homology with HuIFN-α	80–95%	30–50%	<10%

[a] Most subtypes.

least a dozen distinct subtypes of interferon α (IFN-α) [*Brack* et al., 1981; *Goeddel* et al., 1981; *Sehgal* et al., 1981; *Weissmann,* 1981], at least one IFN-β [*Weissenbach* et al., 1980; *Sagar* et al., 1981, 1982], and at least one IFN-γ [*Yip* et al., 1982; *Gray* et al., 1982; *Gray and Goeddel,* 1982]. Most of these genes have now been cloned and sequenced [*Weissmann,* 1981; *Goeddel* et al., 1981; *Gray and Goeddel,* 1982; *Mantei and Weissmann,* 1982; *Pestka* et al., 1982]. Some of the basic physicochemical properties of the three antigenically and chemically distinct types (α, β, γ) are set out in table II.

It is generally assumed that interferon constitutes the first line of defense against viral infection in man and other animals [review: *Sonnenfeld and Merigan,* 1979]. Recovery is certainly delayed, or thwarted altogether, if anti-interferon antibodies are injected [*Virelizier and Gresser,* 1978], or in animals lacking the gene(s) responsible for high-level interferon production [*de Maeyer and de Maeyer-Guignard,* 1979, 1980] or for interferon sensitivity of particular viruses [*Haller* et al., 1980, 1981].

In recent years it has also become evident that interferons are in reality a family of hormones exerting a remarkable array of biological effects in addition to their antiviral role [reviews: *Gresser,* 1977; *de Maeyer and de Maeyer-Guignard,* 1979; *Taylor-Papadimitriou,* 1980; *Vilček* et al., 1980]. Indeed, many people now believe that their principal natural role

Table III. Some biological effects of interferons

1. Inhibition of multiplication of viruses	
2. Inhibition of cell division	
In vitro:	normal and malignant cells in culture
In vivo:	regenerating liver
	bone marrow
	neonatal mouse
	cancer in animals and man
3. Changes in plasma membrane	
Histocompatibility antigens increased	
β-Microglobulin increased	
F_C receptors increased	
Lectin binding increased	
Negative charge increased	
Release of murine leukemia virus decreased	
Cell motility decreased	
Organization of microfilaments and fibronectin disturbed	
4. Immunomodulation	
B cell:	antibody production decreased or increased
T cell:	proliferation suppressed
	lymphokine release enhanced
T_D and/or T_{Sd} cell:	delayed hypersensitivity decreased or increased
T_C cell:	cytotoxicity increased
NK cell:	maturation, recycling and cytotoxicity increased
Macrophage:	activated

may be the regulation of cell growth and differentiation. It is not germane to discuss these particular properties of interferons in any detail in a review on antiviral agents, but they are summarized in table III. They can be seen to fall under three main headings: inhibition of cell division, changes in the plasma membrane and cytoskeleton, and modulation of the immune response [see *Mims and White,* 1984, for fuller treatment].

Though interferons inhibit the growth of malignant cells in vitro as well as in vivo [review: *Gresser and Tovey,* 1978], the multiplication of normal cells in culture is just as susceptible [*Balkwill,* 1979]. The anti-cancer activity of interferon in animals [review: *Gresser and Tovey,* 1978] and in man [review: *Merigan,* 1981a] may be attributable rather to the activation of natural killer (NK) cells [*Gidlund* et al., 1978; *Trinchieri and*

Santoli, 1978; *Reid* et al., 1981], macrophages [*Schultz* et al., 1977], and cytotoxic T (T_c) cells [*Lindahl* et al., 1972]. The immunomodulatory effects of interferons [reviews: *Gresser,* 1977; *Johnson and Baron,* 1977; *de Maeyer and de Maeyer-Guignard,* 1979, 1980] are complex. Whereas the cytotoxicity of various types of effector cell may be enhanced, the replication of lymphocytes may be inhibited, leading to suppression of various arms of the immune response [*Sonnenfeld* et al., 1978; *de Maeyer and de Maeyer-Guignard,* 1979, 1980; *Kadish* et al., 1980; *Kimchi* et al., 1981; *Knop* et al., 1982]. Insofar as IFN-α and -γ are produced by lymphocytes – indeed, IFN-γ is produced only by lymphocytes, following antigen-specific or nonspecific (mitogenic) stimulation [*Epstein,* 1981; *Vilček* et al., 1981] –, these molecules can also be properly regarded as lymphokines [*de Weck* et al., 1980; *Mozes* et al., 1981], induced principally though not exclusively by virus infection and playing a key role in the regulation of the immunological response.

A complete understanding of the immunomodulatory, growth-inhibitory and antiviral activities of interferons will require detailed analysis of the effects of purified preparations of each cloned IFN subtype, preferably on cloned populations of fully characterized lymphocytes and other cells. Already there is some evidence that the three interferon types [*Rubin and Gupta,* 1980] and several cloned subtypes [*Pestka* et al., 1982] may differ significantly in their relative efficacy as immunomodulatory, growth-inhibitory and antiviral agents. Such differences between cloned interferons, or even hybrid or other artificial molecules created by genetic engineering [*Streuli* et al., 1981] or chemical synthesis, could be exploited in the future to target antiviral or anticancer therapy on particular diseases, while minimizing undesirable side effects.

B. Assay of Interferon

Since interferon is defined in terms of its antiviral property it is this biological activity that forms the basis of the classical assays [*Stewart,* 1979; *Pestka,* 1981; *Finter* et al., 1984]. Interferon is titrated for its ability to block multiplication of virus in cultured cells, the endpoint usually being read by plaque reduction, inhibition of CPE, or reduction in virus yield. In view of the relative species specificity of certain IFNs, cells derived from the homologous species are the logical choice, e.g., a diploid strain of human fibroblasts for the assay of HuIFN. However, since HuIFN-α (but not β or γ) subtypes happen to be at least as effective in bovine cells, they are conveniently assayed in the continuous cell line, MDBK [*Rubinstein* et al., 1981]. RNA viruses of the togavirus, rhabdovirus, picornavirus and orthomyxovirus families, being very sensitive to IFN and also fast-growing, are preferred for challenge; traditional choices are Sindbis, vesicular stomatitis virus (VSV), encephalomyocarditis virus (EMC), and influenza. The specific activity of the IFN preparation is expressed in units per milligram of protein, with reference to international standard preparations of known potency [*World Health Organization,* 1982].

Of course, any other biological activity of IFN may also be assayed, e.g., anti-proliferative activity by inhibition of multiplication of the human lymphoblastoid Daudi cell line, or of hemopoietic colony formation by human bone marrow cells [*Pestka* et al., 1981].

In all likelihood, sensitive radioimmunoassays and enzyme-linked immunoassays utilizing monoclonal antibodies known to be specific for a particular IFN or to cross-react with others of the same class [*Secher,* 1981; *Staehelin* et al., 1981b] will rapidly become standard, though of course biological assays will always be needed, especially since synergism between different IFNs has been demonstrated to occur [*Fleischmann,* 1982].

C. Induction and Regulation of Interferon Production

Virtually all viruses are capable of inducing production of interferon α or β, but RNA viruses are in general superior. The togaviruses (e.g., Chikungunya), paramyxoviruses [e.g., Newcastle disease virus (NDV) and Sendai], and reoviruses (which of course contain dsRNA) are particularly good. It is not essential that the virus multiply; indeed, interferon may be produced in cells that are nonpermissive for the virus in question, or with virus whose infectivity has been inactivated by heat or ultraviolet light. Some cytocidal viruses that shut down host cell mRNA and protein synthesis induce more interferon if UV-inactivated (e.g., NDV).

Subsequent to *Isaacs and Lindenmann's* [1957] original discovery it became clear that interferon could be induced by many agents other than viruses. The list is long [*Stringfellow,* 1980b] and includes bacteria, endotoxins, mitogens and a variety of other substances. Notably effective is dsRNA [*Marcus,* 1982], whether naturally occurring, as with the reoviruses, or a totally synthetic polynucleotide, such as polyinosinic acid:polycytidylic acid (polyI.polyC) [*Torrence and de Clercq,* 1977]. Now that monoclonal antibodies against each human IFN are available, it is important to reassess the earlier findings in order to determine which molecular species of IFN are being induced by some of the more unusual agents on the list.

1. Priming

The yield of IFN-α or -β can be considerably enhanced by 'priming' the cells with a low dose of IFN before induction. A typical regime is IFN (100 units/ml) 16 h prior to induction by polyI.polyC [*Stewart,* 1979; *de Maeyer and de Maeyer-Guignard,* 1979]. The mechanism of priming is not understood.

2. Hyporesponsiveness

By contrast, accumulation of a high concentration of intracellular IFN shuts off further IFN synthesis. Moreover, the cell becomes refractory to further induction. This constitutes a major impediment to prolonged production of IFN in vitro, as well as to repeated administration of IFN inducers in vivo; hyporesponsiveness lasts up to 1 week after administration of polyI.polyC in man. Again the mechanism is not understood, but does not appear to be attributable to direct negative feedback by IFN of its own synthesis [*Torrence and de Clercq,* 1977; *de Maeyer and de Maeyer-Guignard,* 1979; *Sehgal* et al., 1981].

3. Superinduction

Assuming that a repressor of interferon synthesis is indeed induced by high concentrations of newly synthesized IFN, early IFN workers, notably *Vilček* and colleagues [1976] demonstrated that the expected shutoff of IFN synthesis could be forestalled by timely administration of inhibitors of protein and mRNA synthesis. A typical protocol is as follows: cycloheximide at the time of induction with polyI.polyC, followed 5 h later by actinomycin D; IFN harvested at 30 h. Known as 'superinduction', this procedure augments the yield of IFN by up to 10-fold (following polyI.polyC, but not viral induction). Although the phenomenon may be plausibly attributed to inhibition of synthesis of the putative repressor (and its mRNA) after the mRNA for IFN has been given time to accumulate but before a sufficient concentration of IFN has been made to induce the repressor, proof is still lacking [*Vilček* et al., 1976; *Torrence and de Clercq,* 1977; *de Maeyer and de Maeyer-Guignard,* 1979; *Sehgal* et al., 1981].

4. Gamma Interferon (IFN-γ)

Wheelock [1965] described a novel type of interferon, produced only by lymphocytes, induced not by viruses but by lectins. It was subsequently discovered that this 'type II' interferon could be induced not only by a wide range of mitogens, but also by allogeneic cells, monoclonal antibodies binding to T-cell surface markers, or specific antigens binding to T lymphocytes previously 'sensitized' (primed) by that particular antigen [reviews: *Epstein,* 1981; *Vilček* et al., 1981]. Accordingly, 'type II interferon' became known also as 'immune interferon'. Both names have now been discarded in favor of 'IFN-γ'.

D. Production of Interferon

1. Leukocyte Interferon (LeIFN)

Leukocytes, particularly lymphocytes, but also macrophages, produce larger quantities of IFN than any other cells. For many years, most of the world's supply of HuIFN came from the laboratory of Dr. *K. Cantell* in Finland, who developed the following method of producing the material from leukocytes. The 'buffy coat' cells collected from donated blood were induced with the paramyxovirus, Sendai, to produce HuIFN-α, which was then concentrated from the supernatant by fractional precipitation at particular pH values [*Cantell* et al., 1981]. The procedure is essentially simple but very costly, the maximum yield from each liter of donated blood being only about 10^7 international units (IU) of HuIFN-α of about 1% purity. The use of leukocytes from leukemia patients [*Pestka* et al., 1981] has the same limitations. Though much of our knowledge of the clinical value of IFN is based on trials conducted with *Cantell's* material, this method of production is clearly incapable of supplying the huge potential market.

2. Lymphoblastoid Interferon

Much greater yields of HuIFN-α can be obtained from continuous lines of lymphoblastoid cells, such as the B-cell line, Namalwa, derived from a Burkitt lymphoma. Such cells can be grown in suspension on an industrial scale in 3,500-liter tanks. Most or all species of HuIFN-α and smaller amounts of -β are present in the product, which is 80% pure and from which Epstein-Barr (EB) virus DNA has been rigorously excluded [*Finter,* 1982].

3. Fibroblast Interferon (F-IFN)

Fibroblasts, by contrast, produce mainly IFN-β (exclusively so when polyI.polyC, rather than virus, is used as inducer [*Vilček* et al., 1981]). The technique of superinduction is often used to enhance the yield. Human diploid strains grow well in monolayer culture but not in suspension. This imposes a serious limitation on large-scale commercial production [*Leong and Horoszewicz,* 1981; *van Damme and Billiau,* 1981] which has been only partially overcome by growing the fibroblast monolayers on the surface of tiny beads ('micro-carriers') in suspension [*Edy* et al., 1982].

4. Gamma Interferon (IFN-γ)

HuIFN-γ is not produced in particularly large amounts following the standard induction protocol (exposure of lymphocytes to mitogen). However, *Yip* et al. [1982] were able to enhance phytohemagglutinin-induced HuIFN-γ production 20-fold by addition of the diterpene ester, 12-O-tetradecanoylphorbol-13-acetate (TPA). The resulting yields from leukocyte concentrates obtained as a by-product of plateletpheresis were just sufficient for partial purification and characterization of the product.

5. Cloning

Recombinant DNA technology has revolutionized the study of interferons, as it has so many other fields. In 1980 a major breakthrough was achieved by *Nagata* et al. [1980], and shortly thereafter by *Goeddel* et al. [1980b], when the gene for a human IFN-α was cloned and expressed in *Escherichia coli* [reviews: *Weissmann,* 1981; *Weissmann* et al., 1982; *Pestka* et al., 1981; *Pestka,* 1983].

In brief, the strategy pursued by *Nagata* et al. [1980] was as follows. Messenger RNA from interferon-producing human leukocytes was subjected to rate zonal centrifugation, and the fractions were tested for their capacity to produce IFN-α in frog *(Xenopus)* oocytes. The most active fraction was used as template for the transcription of cDNA, which was then inserted into the plasmid pBR322, thence to *E. coli.* Numerous transformed colonies were then screened for plasmid DNA containing IFN-specific sequences, using a hybridization translation assay of IFN mRNA in oocytes. A plasmid containing a somewhat abbreviated IFN cDNA insert was detected and employed as a probe in a more extensive search, which resulted in the isolation of a clone of *E. coli* constitutively synthesizing IFN that displayed antiviral activity in human cells.

Basically similar approaches were employed to clone human IFN-β genes in *E. coli* [*Derynck* et al., 1980; *Goeddel* et al., 1980a; *Taniguchi* et al., 1980a], and again the bacteria synthesized interferon. Most recently, the HuIFN-γ gene has been cloned [*Gray* et al., 1982]. This is an important development because IFN-γ, which has proved difficult to produce in any quantity by alternative methods, is widely believed to be a more potent and/or selective immunoregulatory and anticancer molecule than either of the other two types.

The rather low yields of interferon obtained with the earliest protocol [*Nagata* et al., 1980] were improved up to 10,000-fold by the use of expression plasmids containing appropriate prokaryotic promoters [*Goeddel* et al., 1980a, b; *Weissmann,* 1981; *Yelverton* et al., 1981]. For example, cloning of the IFN gene in a plasmid containing the *trp* promoter allows the transformed clone of bacteria to be grown to high density in the presence of tryptophan to suppress the expression of the gene, then switched to tryptophan-free medium to derepress IFN synthesis [*Goeddel* et al., 1980b].

The yields of interferon so obtained ($1-2 \times 10^8$ units, i.e., 0.3–0.7 mg IFN per liter of bacterial culture, and now up to 10 mg) are vastly greater than those obtained from leukocyte, lymphoblastoid or fibroblast cultures. Overall, it is estimated that the cost of production of commercial interferon should be reduced by up to 100-fold as a result of recombinant DNA technology.

Potentially, costs may be even further reduced by commercial exploitation of the cloning of IFN genes in yeasts, which have been grown industrially in inexpensive medium for many years, and which, like other eukaryotic cells, are able to glycosylate IFN-β and -γ. The gene for human LeIF-D (IFN-α_1) was cloned in *Saccharomyces cerevisiae* in a plasmid capable of autonomous replication and selection in both yeast and *E. coli* [*Hitzeman* et al., 1981]. Although yields were only about 2×10^6 units of IFN per liter of culture, it was predicted that further genetic manipulation would bring about substantial improvement.

Most recently, the gene for HuIFN-γ has been cloned in mammalian cells by *Gray* et al. [1982]. An SV40 vector was used to transfect an SV40-transformed monkey kidney cell line, COS-7; HuIFN-γ was synthesized, glycosylated and secreted by these cells. Shortly thereafter, *Mantei and Weissmann* [1982] reported the successful cloning of the gene for HuIFNα_1 in mouse L cells.

6. Chemical Synthesis

A further major achievement during this dramatic few months was the chemical synthesis of the complete gene for human interferon γ_1 by *Edge* et al. [1981]. This represents by far the largest gene to be synthesized to this date, and the first using the solid-phase phosphodiester method for the synthesis of oligonucleotides; no fewer than 67 separate oligonucleotides were constructed then enzymatically ligated to produce the 514 base-pair molecule. Initiation and termination signals plus restriction endonuclease sites for plasmid insertion were included, so that the synthetic gene could be cloned and expressed in *E. coli.* Furthermore, the actual nucleotide sequence of this human gene was modified to optimize the use of codons most commonly preferred for high-level expression in bacteria.

This technology opens up the possibility of synthesizing artificial IFN genes, perhaps shorter than the original, coding for those segments of the IFN molecule bearing the active site(s) for desired antiviral, anti-proliferative or immunoregulatory functions. Analysis of hybrid interferons produced by cloning recombinant cDNA molecules created by ligating segments derived from different IFN cDNAs that have been cleaved at common restriction endonuclease sites [*Streuli* et al., 1981] may shed some light on such structure-activity relationships.

At the time of writing, the protein itself had not been synthesized chemically, but substantial portions of the interferon molecule had been synthesized by the Merrifield procedure.

E. Purification of Interferon

Human interferons α and β have now been purified to homogeneity following production in human cells, or in bacteria by recombinant DNA technology. In the latter case, IFN is not transported out of the cell, which is a mixed blessing; on the one hand, it means that the bacteria must be lysed to release the IFN then care taken to remove endotoxins and to prevent degradation of the product by proteases; on the other, it facilitates initial concentration by a simple centrifugation step.

Many of the classical techniques for protein fractionation by precipitation, affinity chromatography, gel filtration, and SDS-polyacrylamide gel electrophoresis (PAGE) were used to obtain partial purification during the mid-70s [reviews: *Berg,* 1982; *Stewart,* 1979; *Knight and Fahey,* 1981; *Pestka,* 1981; 1983]. Two particular properties of interferons were generally exploited. The acid stability of IFN-α and -β enabled contaminating proteins to be denatured by prolonged exposure at pH 2. Secondly, the fact that IFN-β and -γ are glycoproteins meant that they could be absorbed onto lectin columns. However, persuasive evidence of purification to homogeneity had to await the application of high-performance liquid chromatography [*Rubinstein* et al., 1979; review: *Pestka* et al., 1981] and immunoaffinity chromatography [*Zoon* et al., 1979]. Monoclonal antibodies were introduced for the latter purpose by *Secher and Burke* [1980] and *Staehelin* et al. [1981a]. Single bands of protein on SDS-PAGE have now been obtained by several groups, and HuIFN-α has been crystallized [*Weissmann,* 1981; *Miller* et al., 1982]. The latter development should pave the way for determination of the tertiary structure by X-ray crystallography.

The specific activity of purified HuIFN-α and -β appears to be in the order of $(2-4) \times 10^8$ units per milligram of protein [*Pestka* et al., 1981], though *Gresser* et al. [1979] reported a figure of 2×10^9 units per milligram for MuIFN-α.

HuIFN-γ has proved much more difficult to purify, as it is produced by mitogen-induced lymphocytes in unsatisfactory quantity, and, by contrast with IFN-α and -β, is labile at pH 2, denatured by SDS (0.1%), indeed somewhat more labile generally [*Vilček* et al., 1981]. Partial purification was achieved by *Yip* et al. [1982], but definitive characterization became possible only following production of HuIFN-γ by recombinant DNA technology by *Gray* and colleagues [*Gray* et al., 1982; *Gray and Goeddel,* 1982].

F. Chemical Structure of Human Interferons and Their Genes

The compilation of IFN cDNA libraries, which in turn were used as probes to screen human chromosomal DNA, soon revealed that there are at least a dozen distinct human genes coding for a family of related interferons of the α type [*Nagata* et al., 1980; *Taniguchi* et al., 1980b; *Goeddel* et al., 1980b, 1981; *Allen and Fantes,* 1980; *Brack* et al., 1981; *Weissmann,* 1981; *Weissmann* et al., 1982] and a less closely related β_1 [*Derynck* et al., 1980; *Goeddel* et al., 1980a; *Taniguchi* et al., 1980b]. Homology between subtypes within the human α family is 80(–95)% if the cDNA sequence coding for the more variable signal peptide is ignored; approximately 60% of the amino acids in the deduced sequence of the mature IFN-α molecules occur in invariant positions [*Goeddel* et al., 1981]. On the other hand, homology between the cDNAs for α and β_1 IFNs is only 30(–50)%, with 23% of amino acids occupying identical positions. Tertiary structure is maintained in part by four highly conserved cysteines, forming two intramolecular disulfide bonds, between residues 1–98 and 29–138.

Most of the mature HuIFN-α subtypes, as well as β_1, consist of precisely 166 amino acids (mol.wt. 19,000 daltons), following the removal of a 21–23 amino acid signal peptide. In human cells, but not in bacteria, an additional 10 amino acids are presumably removed by post-translational cleavage from the COOH-terminus, for the three HuIFN-α subtypes purified from human leukemic cells and sequenced by *Levy* et al. [1981] were lacking these 10 residues predicted from the cDNA sequences.

In addition to the genes described above, there appear to be a number of pseudogenes. One such pseudogene, described by *Goeddel* et al. [1981], contains a single additional nucleotide, with the result that termination codons occur downstream; others contain several insertions and/or deletions [*Weissmann*, 1981]. Furthermore, there are several allelic variants. Minor differences may occur between essentially similar IFN subtypes produced by different cell types. For instance, Genentech's major human leukocyte interferon subtype LeIFN-A (otherwise known as IFLrA) contains one less amino acid than does Biogen's IFN α-2 and differs in a number of other residues. It is premature, therefore, to attempt to equate the various cloned IFNs produced by different laboratories, and certainly too early to assume that the products of all HuIFN genes have been identified.

The truth of this assertion is borne out by the recent description of additional human α and β interferons of somewhat higher Mr, which are perhaps under separate control and not normally made in large amounts. First, *Weissenbach* et al. [1980] and *Sagar* et al. [1981] discovered HuIFN-β_2, which is somewhat larger than, and shows relatively little homology with β_1; then *Sagar* et al. [1982] postulated the existence of β_3, β_4 and β_5 on the basis of their finding five 'translationally active' HuIFN-β mRNA species in polyI.polyC-induced fibroblasts. These additional β-IFNs are not to be confused with the dimeric form of HuIFN-β_1 (mol.wt. 40,000) described by *Knight and Fahey* [1981]. Additional subtypes of HuIFN-α, designated α_L because of their large size, were recently discovered by *Sehgal* et al. [1981]; they display very little homology with the previously described smaller ('α_S') subtypes which all fall within the Mr range 16,000–21,000 as determined by SDS-PAGE [*Pestka* et al., 1981].

Recent evidence also indicates the existence of acid(pH 2)-labile interferon(s) α secreted by immune lymphocytes [*Grundy* et al., 1982; *Balkwill* et al., 1983]. Such acid-labile α-interferons have been found in patients with the 'gay lymphadenopathy syndrome' and the acquired immune deficiency syndrome (AIDS) [*DeStefano* et al., 1982] or certain autoimmune syndromes, notably lupus erythematosus [*Preble* et al., 1982], but the significance of these associations is unknown.

Partially purified HuIFN-γ resolved on SDS-PAGE into two peaks of apparent Mr 20,000 and 25,000, both of which displayed antiviral activity, were glycoproteins, labile at pH 2, and failed to react with anti-IFN-α or anti-IFN-β serum [*Yip* et al., 1982]. The authors postulated that these are two subtypes of HuIFN-γ, but it is also quite possible that they represent differently cleaved or glycosylated forms of the same gene-product [*Gray and Goeddel,* 1982]. The much higher Mr forms previously described [*Vilček* et al., 1981; *Epstein,* 1981] may be multimers arising by spontaneous aggregation. The HuIFN-γ cDNA cloned in *E. coli* by *Gray* et al. [1982] codes for a protein containing 166 amino acids, 20 of which are thought to constitute a signal peptide; the Mr of the cleaved 146 residue molecule was calculated to be 17,110 before glycosylation.

The gene for HuIFN-γ has now been isolated and, unlike the genes for HuIFN-α and -β, shown to contain introns, three in number, as well as a repetitive DNA element [*Gray and Goeddel,* 1982]. The gene displays virtually no relationship to those for the known HuIFN-α or -β subtypes, except for some homology with a conserved region of IFN-α and the fact that 12% of individual amino acids are in comparable positions.

At the time of writing, the three-dimensional structure of interferon had not been determined by X-ray crystallography, but *Sternberg and Cohen* [1982] had predicted from amino acid sequences that the molecule contains four α-helices packed into a right-handed bundle, while *Wetzel* et al. [1982] had used an algorithm to conclude also that both α and β IFNs are highly helical globular proteins with a densely packed hydrophobic core.

Table II summarizes some of the properties characterizing the three known types of human interferon.

G. Antiviral Action of Interferon

Over the past decade the fascinating story of the presumed mechanisms of action of interferon – or, to express it more cautiously, the biochemical consequences of interferon's action – has unfolded [reviews: *Baglioni,* 1979, 1983; *Revel,* 1979; *Cayley* et al., 1981; *Lengyel,* 1981, 1982; *Lebleu and Content,* 1982]. These biochemical events have turned out to be unexpectedly intricate, involving the induction by interferon of no fewer than three separate enzymes and a further requirement for dsRNA in their activation. Yet, as will become evident later, we cannot assume that the story is yet complete, or even correct, intellectually satisfying though it may appear to be.

1. Binding of Interferon and Induction of Enzymes

Interferons α and β bind to a common interferon receptor on the cell surface [*Aguet,* 1980]; the receptor for IFN-γ seems to be distinct [*Branca and Baglioni,* 1981]. By a process that is completely unknown and may or may not require interferon to enter the cell, binding of a very small number of molecules is sufficient to trigger the synthesis of at least half a dozen proteins detectable by gel electrophoresis [*Rubin and Gupta,* 1980], and an additional set in the case of IFN-γ [*Weil* et al., 1983]. The antiviral state does not develop if mRNA or protein synthesis is blocked by inhibitors. Three induced enzymes are first detectable intracellularly within 2–6 h and reach peak levels within 15–30 h [*Baglioni,* 1979; *Revel,* 1979; *Lengyel,* 1982]. These enzymes, 2-5A synthetase, RNase L, and protein kinase have been fully characterized and postulated to be instrumental in implementing the antiviral action of IFN [*Baglioni,* 1979, 1983; *Cayley* et al., 1981; *Lengyel,* 1981, 1982].

Two of these enzymes require dsRNA for their activation. Such dsRNA is presumed to be formed as an intermediate or by-product in the replication of all RNA and DNA viruses, though it must be said that the evidence for this is lacking, especially for DNA viruses [*Baglioni,* 1982]. *Nilsen and Baglioni* [1979] presented some evidence to support a hypothesis that cellular RNA may tend to be spared while viral RNA is degraded by the IFN-induced 2-5A synthetase/RNase L system because 2-5A, hence 2-5A-activated RNase L, will be present in highest concentration in the immediate vicinity of the viral ds replicative intermediate (and of viral mRNA containing ds regions). It is interesting that dsRNA appears to be essential both for the induction of IFN and for the subsequent activation of two of the three IFN-induced enzymes. While IFN alone can prepare the ground for the inhibition of protein synthesis by inducing the production of the requisite enzymes in inactive form, uninfected cells are not destroyed because final establishment of the antiviral state must await activation of these enzymes by dsRNA which can only be provided by viral infection.

2. 2-5A Synthetase

Kerr and his colleagues in England were principally responsible for opening up this Pandora's box of enzymes with their discovery that, in the presence of dsRNA, protein synthesis was inhibited in cell-free extracts from interferon-pretreated cells [*Kerr* et al., 1974; *Roberts* et al., 1976]. Subsequently, they identified the inhibitor as ppp A2′p5′A2′p5′A (known as '2-5A' for short) and, furthermore, demonstrated that 2-5A is formed from ATP by an enzyme which they activated by the ingenious technique of absorption to the dsRNA, polyI.polyC on agarose beads [*Kerr and Brown,* 1978].

The enzyme, (2′-5′)$(A)_n$ synthetase, or 2-5A polymerase, which catalyzes the synthesis of 2-5A from ATP, is induced by IFN-α, -β and -γ [*Baglioni,* 1983; *Lengyel,* 1982]. The enzyme has been purified [*Ball,* 1982; *Cayley* et al., 1981; *Lengyel,* 1982]. It is active only when bound to dsRNA. Its products are a family of oligoadenylates of a unique kind.

The compounds designated (2′-5′) oligo(A), or (2′-5′)$(A)_n$, or more strictly, (2′-5′) pppA$(pA)_n$, were shown to be oligonucleotides consisting of short chains of adenosines linked, uniquely, by 2′-5′ phosphodiester bonds (rather than the 3′-5′ bonds found in all natural polynucleotides); the most abundant were di-, tri- and tetra-adenylates, but only trimers and longer oligomers were active [*Kerr and Brown,* 1978]. Though 2-5A has a short half-life, it could be demonstrated in IFN-treated, virus-infected cells. When introduced artificially into cells, 2-5A inhibited protein synthesis, cell division and viral multiplication [*Cayley* et al., 1981], as, incidentally, do certain phosphodiesterase-resistant 2-5A derivatives which could conceivably be developed as antiviral chemotherapeutic agents [*Doetsch* et al., 1981].

3. RNase L

The mechanism of the antiviral action of 2-5A was unravelled as a result of the work of several independent groups. *Lengyel* and his colleagues had observed that, in the presence of dsRNA and ATP, both reovirus mRNA and cellular mRNA were degraded more rapidly in extracts of IFN-treated cells [*Lengyel,* 1982]. Then *Clemens and Williams* [1978] showed that addition of 2-5A to an in vitro protein-synthesizing system reduced the translation of mRNA. *Baglioni* et al. [1978] demonstrated this to be attributable to an endoribonuclease that is activated by 2-5A. The function of 2-5A is, therefore, to bind to the latent endonuclease (RNase L, otherwise known as RNase F), thereby activating the enzyme to destroy both viral and cellular mRNA as well as rRNA and perhaps other cellular RNAs, by specific cleavage on the 3′-side of UpN doublets [*Baglioni,* 1983; *Lengyel,* 1982].

4. Protein Kinase

A second pathway, quite unrelated to 2-5A synthetase/RNase L, is inhibited by interferon in the presence of dsRNA. A dsRNA-dependent protein kinase was found independently by *Lebleu* et al. [1976] and *Roberts* et al. [1976] to phosphorylate at least one protein besides itself (autophosphorylation) in extracts of IFN-treated cells to which dsRNA had been added. This particular protein kinase, which is induced by IFN-α, -β and -γ, was first purified by *Sen* et al. in 1978 [see *Lengyel,* 1982]. The protein phosphorylated by the activated kinase was shown by *Farrell* et al. [1978] to be the α subunit of the eukaryotic peptide chain initiation factor, eIF-2. The phosphorylated eIF-2 is inactive, hence can no longer catalyze the formation of the ternary complex between itself, met-tRNA and GTP.

5. Inhibition of Methylation of Viral mRNA

Inhibition of protein synthesis by IFN may occur by yet another mechanism, namely, inhibition of methylation of viral mRNA. *Sen* et al. [1977] first discovered that a labile inhibitor of methylation of reovirus mRNA is induced in IFN-treated cells. However, as only the 2-O-methylation of the ribose moieties is diminished, the mRNA is translated satisfactorily. Subsequently, *Baglioni's* group demonstrated that VSV mRNA is not translated in IFN-treated cells because in this case the 5′-terminal guanosine 'cap' is unmethylated, apparently as a result of IFN-induced changes in the levels of S-adenosylmethionine and S-adenosylhomocysteine [*Baglioni,* 1983].

6. Other Effects

The pathways to inhibition of viral protein synthesis which were discussed above are set out in diagrammatic form in figure 1. Several additional biochemical changes have been reported to occur in IFN-treated cells [*Baglioni,* 1979, 1983; *Revel,* 1979; *Lengyel,* 1981, 1982]. The antiviral action of IFN against murine leukemia virus, in which the release of budding virions is blocked [*Pitha* et al., 1976; *Friedman,* 1977], may well be secondary to effects of the hormone on the plasma membrane. *Pfeffer* et al. [1980] have described quite marked interferon-induced effects on the structure and function of cells, notably on microfilament organization, fibronectin distribution and cell motility. Furthermore, interferon induces an increase in the intracellular concentration of cyclic GMP, but this does not appear to be central to its antiviral or anticellular action. Several years ago, *Stewart* et al. [1972] made an observation that has yet to be explained, namely that interferon-treated cells acquire increased susceptibility to the cytotoxic effects of the dsRNA, polyI.polyC.

At the moment, it is impossible to apportion the appropriate measure of relevance to the multitude of biochemical effects ascribed to the several (pure or impure) IFNs in the literature. It is clear that IFN is pleiotropic in its effects, and this is consistent with the view of IFN as a hormone, as well as with the teleological argument that the body's principal antiviral agent must have evolved to block viral replication at multiple points in order to forestall the replacement of all natural viruses with IFN-resistant mutants. Nevertheless, it is premature to be dogmatic about which effects are real rather than artefactual, let alone about which are the critical mediators of IFN's antiviral action. We know even less about the biochemical mechanisms of the numerous other effects of the several distinct IFNs to be described below.

7. Postscript

While the several pathways described above (see also fig. 1) could explain the antiviral action of interferons, it is becoming increasingly doubtful that any of them represents the key mechanism [for further discussion see *Baglioni,* 1983; *Ball,* 1982; *Lebleu and Content,* 1982]. Several lines of data are now emerging which demonstrate that the antiviral state created by interferon is not necessarily correlated with the induction of either 2-5A synthetase or the 73K protein kinase. For example, in MRC5 cells interferon causes no rise in the basal level of either enzyme, yet confers resistance to challenge with vesicular stomatitis virus [*Hovanessian* et al., 1980].

Baglioni [1983] contends that the role of the protein kinase as a mediator of interferon action remains to be demonstrated. He cites the facts that (i) the activity of this enzyme increases only 3- to 10-fold following induction, compared with 10- to 10,000-fold generally for 2-5A synthetase; (ii) if phosphorylation of eIF-2 occurs at all in intact cells (as

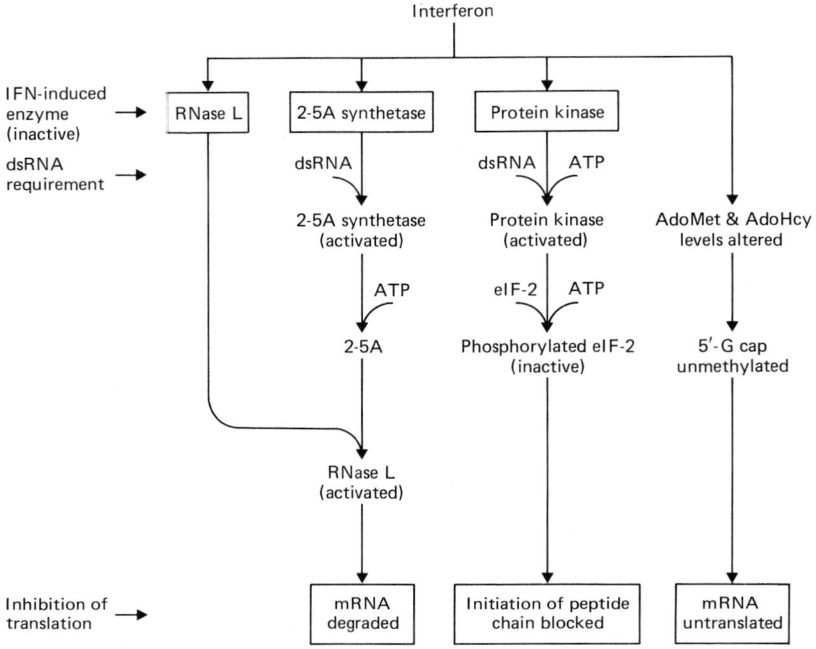

Fig. 1. Antiviral action of interferon: postulated pathways.

opposed to cell extracts), it may be rapidly reversed by the cell's phosphoprotein phosphatase; (iii) it is hard to envisage how eIF-2 could discriminate between viral and cellular protein synthesis.

The postulated role of 2-5A synthetase has also come under fire [*Ball*, 1982]. Basal levels of 2-5A synthetase differ greatly from one cell type to another, some producing high levels of 2-5A synthetase, 2-5A and RNAse L constitutively, in the absence of interferon treatment. The enzyme level is also influenced by such factors as growth rate and hormone treatment [*Kimchi* et al., 1981]. Furthermore, the level of 2-5A itself fluctuates widely with time in normal or IFN-treated cells; this may reflect the level of a phosphodiesterase, found in interferon-treated cell extracts, which degrades 2-5A (and the C-C-A terminus of tRNA) and may thereby regulate interferon's antiviral activity [*Schmidt* et al., 1979]. Perhaps 2-5A synthetase and 2-5A have a natural role quite unrelated to interferon-induced inhibition of viral replication. Their real function may be concerned with regulation of cell growth and differentiation, by activating RNAse L to cleave mRNA$\pm$ribosomal RNA and/or heterogeneous nuclear RNA [*Cayley* et al., 1981; *Lengyel,* 1982]. *Ball* [1982] argues that not only is there no evidence of any selectivity of RNAse L for viral mRNA (as opposed to cellular RNA) but neither is there persuasive evidence that breakdown of viral mRNA occurs at an enhanced rate in most interferon-treated virus-infected cells (as opposed to cell extracts).

A further concern is that dsRNA, which is absolutely required for activation of both the 2-5A synthetase/RNAse L pathway and the protein kinase pathway of IFN's antiviral action, has in fact not been demonstrated conclusively to occur in cells infected with DNA viruses, which are not only reasonably satisfactory inducers of IFN synthesis but also fully susceptible to IFN. Indeed, *Nilsen* et al., using a sensitive assay, were unable to detect any dsRNA (or 2-5A) in cells infected with an IFN-sensitive RNA virus, VSV, suggesting that further mediators of IFN action, not dependent on dsRNA, remain to be discovered [see *Baglioni,* 1983].

H. Pharmacology

Most clinical experience of the pharmacokinetics and toxicity of interferon so far has been confined to purified mixed preparations of 'leukocyte' or 'fibroblast' interferons [*Pollard and Merigan,* 1978; *Baron* et al., 1979; *Billiau,* 1981; *Merigan,* 1981a, b], although data are beginning to come in on cloned subtypes [*Gutterman* et al., 1982]. Le-IFN (HuIFN-α) is commonly administered intramuscularly (i.m.), because this route is convenient and ensures a more prolonged and even release of IFN into the bloodstream, allowing serum levels of 50–500 units/ml to be maintained following the usual daily injection of 3×10^6–8×10^7 units. On the other hand, F-IFN (HuIFN-β) has generally been given intravenously (i.v.) because most of it is not detectable in the circulation following i.m. delivery; there is still some debate about whether this reflects destruction of IFN-β in muscle or binding by muscle [*Billiau,* 1981]. But the half-life of both IFN-α and -β is quite short following i.v. inoculation. Degradation occurs mainly in the kidney and liver. Relatively little (approximately 3%) of any IFN type crosses the blood-brain barrier into the CSF, but it has been administered intrathecally [*Jacobs* et al., 1981]. It is not effective by mouth. Following intranasal delivery it is rapidly swept away by ciliary movement of mucus. Topical application to the eye is reliable. Recent successes with the treatment of cancer by local injection into the tumor itself suggest that this and other forms of topical delivery such as slow release from liposomes, or conjugation to an antibody or other targeting molecule, should be explored further.

Toxic side effects are regularly observed, and may be marked with doses in excess of 10^7 units per day, even when highly purified cloned IFN subtypes are employed [reviews: *Merigan,* 1981a; *Scott* et al., 1981; *Gutterman* et al., 1982; *World Health Organization,* 1982]. Fever is standard at high dosage, but lasts only a day or so. Severe fatigue is the most debilitating symptom and may be accompanied by malaise, anorexia, myalgia, headache, nausea, vomiting, weight loss, erythema, and tenderness at the injection site, partial alopecia (reversible), dry mouth, reversible peripheral sensory neuropathy or CNS signs. The incidence of peripheral neuritis was so unacceptably high in a recent clinical trial in which interferon was used in combination with adenine arabinoside that the study had to be terminated. Various indicators of bone marrow suppression (granulocytopenia, thrombocytopenia, leukopenia), reversible on cessation of therapy, are regularly observed if high-dose IFN administration is prolonged. Hepatotoxicity, revealed by abnormal liver function tests, is less common and also reversible.

It used to be assumed that interferons were non-immunogenic. Recently however, anti-IFN antibodies have been detected in a small number of patients following the administration of interferon [*Gutterman* et al., 1982]. Now it is apparent that this is not an uncommon development in patients receiving HuIFN (α or β) and, furthermore, that some patients, especially those suffering from autoimmune disease or cancer, can, less commonly, develop low levels of antibody to their own endogenous interferon [*Panem* et al., 1982]. The short- or long-term clinical significance of such antibodies has yet to be evaluated. An important question is whether novel antigenic determinants are exposed on IFNs manufactured by recombinant DNA technology, perhaps as a result of the lack of carbohydrate on those produced in bacteria, or amino acid differences (especially in hybrid IFNs), or atypical disulfide cross-links, etc.

I. Clinical Efficacy

Again, most of the clinical experience with interferon has been with HuLe-IFN (= HuIFN-α) and, to a lesser extent, HuF-IFN (= HuIFN-β), of varying degrees of purity. Many of the trials have been uncontrolled, and some reports are little more than anecdotal. This has raised false expectations – on the stock market as well as in the clinic. Still, well-planned, placebo-controlled, double-blind trials are now being conducted with purified, cloned as well as mixed, interferons. Some modest successes are being obtained, the dosage generally required being in excess of 10^6 units per day (sometimes over 10^8 units per day), although *Scott and Tyrrell* [1980] reported lower doses to be effective. The summary that follows is selective and concentrates on those clinical conditions against which interferon appeared to show at least some real promise at the time of writing [reviews: *Dunnick and Galasso,* 1979, 1980; *Scott and Tyrrell,* 1980; *Merigan,* 1981a, b; *de Maeyer and Schellekens,* 1983; *Baron* et al., 1982; *Came and Carter,* 1983; *Kono,* 1982; *Munk and Kirchner,* 1982; *Pollard,* 1982; *World Health Organization,* 1982; *Finter* et al., 1984].

1. Viral Diseases

One of the great hopes for interferon has always been that it might prove to be the answer to the common cold and other annoying upper respiratory infections, despite the plethora of causal agents. Therefore it came as no surprise that the first moderately encouraging report of the efficacy of interferon in a natural viral infection in man indicated that IFN delivered by intranasal aerosol spray conferred partial protection against rhinovirus-induced colds [*Merigan* et al., 1973]. More recent studies using *E.coli*-cloned HuIFN-α2 have confirmed that colds can be prevented by intranasal installation of IFN in high dosage (total of 10^8 units) at frequent intervals for several days commencing prior to viral challenge [*Scott* et al., 1982]. However, chemoprophylaxis is impracticable; what is required is a 'cure' for the common cold.

High interferon levels are difficult to maintain in the nasopharynx because mucus is removed so rapidly by ciliary action. Cotton pledgets retain the drug for longer, and anti-histamines help slightly, by drying the mucus membrane [*Greenberg* et al., 1982]. Novel methods of delivery may yet have to be devised, but it is essential that they cause no discomfort, if they are to be marketable for the treatment of so trivial a complaint as the common cold.

Interferon may have a role to play in the treatment of certain other viral diseases, notably those caused by the herpesviruses, hepatitis viruses and papillomaviruses.

Oddly enough, though herpesviruses are not notably sensitive to interferon in cell culture, they respond quite well in vivo. In 1978, *Merigan* and colleagues demonstrated in a controlled trial that HuLe-IFN at 3.5×10^7 units per day limited somewhat the progression and dissemination of vesicles, the severity of symptoms and the duration of post-herpetic neuralgia in cancer patients suffering from cutaneous herpes zoster [*Merigan,* 1981a,b]. Merigan's group also reported modest success with varicella in children with cancer. HuIFN-α has also been reported to reduce the incidence of mucocutaneous herpes simplex following surgery for trigeminal neuralgia. The results of current trials against genital herpes are awaited with interest. Herpetic keratoconjunctivitis (dendritic ulcer of the cornea) can be treated more effectively with a combination of interferon and trifluorothymidine than with either alone. There is also evidence that reactivation of cytomegalovirus (CMV) and the accompanying disease that follows immunosuppression, e.g., for renal transplantation, is reduced by interferon [*Hirsch* et al., 1983]. Infectious mononucleosis is a common, debilitating disease for which specific chemotherapy is needed, but no beneficial effect of interferon has yet been reported. Nor does it seem to have any effect on the congenital CMV infection, cytomegalic inclusion disease [*Stiehm* et al., 1982].

Both chronic active hepatitis B and the asymptomatic hepatitis B carrier state are amenable to prolonged treatment with high doses of HuIFN-α or -β. A marked decline in viral DNA polymerase activity in the serum is the most regular indicator of a positive response, but a fall in HBeAg, HBcAg, HBsAg, and Dane particles may also be detectable, as may restoration of near-normal titers in biochemical tests of liver function. Unfortunately, such remissions usually last only as long as IFN therapy is continued. Better results are obtained with a schedule of treatment in which interferon is alternated with adenine arabinoside in multiple cycles extending over several months [*Scullard* et al., 1981]. Virus was cleared from the serum of about half the patients with chronic active, or chronic persistent, hepatitis treated in this way, but the incidence of peripheral neuritis and other manifestations of neurotoxicity [*Sacks* et al., 1982] were so high in a more extensive trial that it had to be terminated.

Perhaps the most spectacular results so far have been reported with juvenile laryngeal papilloma, a severe recurrent viral condition calling for repeated surgical removal. Again, however, the (benign) tumors tend to recur when therapy is withdrawn. HuIFN-α and -β have also been used successfully to treat other types of human viral papilloma, including verruca vulgaris (the common wart) and condyloma acuminata (genital warts) [*Pazin* et al., 1982].

Romano et al. [1980] reported that HuIFN-β, delivered topically to patients with epidemic keratoconjunctivitis (assumed, but proven in only a minority, to be due to adenovirus type 8), considerably reduced the severity and duration of the disease; this work awaits confirmation [*Sundmacher,* 1982]. More extensive trials are now underway to ascertain the efficacy of various interferons against eye infections caused by enterovirus 70 and coxsackie A24, as well as adenoviruses.

Interferon has also been shown to be very effective in protecting animals after challenge with rabies virus [*Plotkin,* 1980] and is now under trial in man. Many other lethal viral diseases of man, such as the encephalitides and the hemorrhagic fevers, are potentially vulnerable to interferon therapy; clinical trials are in progress against some of the more exotic zoonoses, such as Ebola. Studies have also been initiated to determine the response to IFN of certain chronic viral infections, including major diseases of currently unknown etiology, such as multiple sclerosis (MS). In a small uncontrolled trial, *Jacobs* et al. [1981] claimed that MS patients treated with HuIFN-β intrathecally responded with diminished frequency of exacerbations; much larger, double-blind, trials extending over several years will be necessary to evaluate therapeutic efficacy in a disease so notorious for spontaneous fluctuations in the patient's clinical state.

Table IV lists those viral diseases against which HuIFN appears to have displayed at least some activity so far; the list is certain to be obsolete by the time this monograph is published.

2. Cancer

Strander [1977] precipitated a flurry of excitement in cancer circles and even on Wall Street when he reported encouraging but preliminary results of a long-term HuIFN-α trial initiated years earlier on osteosarcoma in Sweden. *Strander* also claimed promising results with multiple myeloma and Hodgkin's disease, then other groups extended his findings to embrace acute leukemia as well. Partial regression of metastatic breast carcinoma as well as multiple myeloma and malignant (non-Hodgkin's) lymphoma was reported in an uncontrolled pilot study using Le-IFN by *Gutterman* et al. [1980], and extended using 'recombinant' HuLe-IFN (IFNrA) to include renal carcinoma and certain others [*Gutterman* et al., 1982]. A Yugoslavian team published results of a preliminary study indicating that crude HuLe-IFN administered by injection directly into the

Table IV. Antiviral activity of interferons in man

Virus	Disease	Route[1]
Rhinovirus	common cold	i.n.
Herpes simplex	keratitis	ocular
	herpes facialis, genitalis	i.m.
Varicella-zoster	herpes zoster	i.m.
	varicella	
Cytomegalovirus	activation in immunosuppressed?	i.m.
Hepatitis B	chronic active or carrier	i.m., i.v.
Papilloma	laryngeal papilloma	local
	warts (common or genital)	
Adenovirus	keratoconjunctivitis?	ocular

[1] i.n. = Intranasal; i.m. = intramuscular; i.v. = intravenous; local = injected into lesion.

cancer produced 'complete or partial regressions for up to 6 months' of malignant papillomatosis of the bladder and malignant melanoma as well as breast carcinoma [*Ikič* et al., 1981]. More recently, local injection of HuIFN-α into gliomas and medulloblastomas of the brain, and into malignant melanomas and squamous and basal cell carcinomas of the skin is said to have led to complete or partial regression in a substantial proportion of the patients so treated [*World Health Organization,* 1982]. It must be added, however, that several other carefully conducted trials have given less encouraging results [e.g., see *Munk and Kirchner,* 1982].

3. Perspective

It is too early to be dogmatic about the value of interferons in the treatment of viral infections or cancer. The euphoria of the late 1970s has been supplanted by a more cautious, balanced belief that interferons, while no panacea, may nevertheless come to occupy an important though limited place in both antiviral and anticancer chemotherapy. Presently, it appears that interferons have a demonstrable effect on a number of viral diseases, notably those due to papillomaviruses, herpesviruses, and hepatitis B virus, and that they may have a future against additional diseases if suitable protocols can be developed for timely delivery of the appropriate interferon by the appropriate route. On the other hand, results so far are not sufficiently impressive to conclude that interferon should be preferred over newer antiviral agents to be discussed below.

The situation regarding cancer is more complex. As of now, it does seem that a small minority of patients with certain types of cancer respond favorably to vigorous interferon therapy with some sort of remission or partial regression, always temporary. In several instances this is no more than can be achieved with other modern chemotherapeutic agents; in others, it may represent the best or only hope available at this juncture.

While some regard the whole interferon saga as a kind of bad dream from which we shall soon awaken to find that nothing is really there, others believe that we have barely scraped the surface so far. Much more work is now needed to test the effects of very high doses of pure preparations of each HuIFN subtype, as well as of mixed pure interferons α, β and γ, and of mixtures reconstituted from cloned subtypes. In all likelihood it will be discovered that particular subtypes are considerably more potent than others, and/or 'specialize' in different antiviral, anti-proliferative or immunomodulatory properties [*Rubin and Gupta,* 1980; *Pestka* et al., 1982] which can be exploited for the specific chemotherapy of particular viral, neoplastic, or indeed additional types of disease. Nor is it inconceivable that, by recombining cDNAs of different IFN subtypes [*Weissmann* et al., 1982; *Pestka* et al., 1982] or synthesizing novel cDNAs [*Edge* et al., 1981], more potent, more stable, less toxic IFNs with particular properties required for specific purposes may be tailor-made for the treatment of individual diseases. Quite minor differences in primary amino acid sequence can markedly alter the antiviral and anticellular spectra, as well as the pharmacological properties of various recIFNs and hybrid IFNs [*Lee* et al., 1982]. Combinations of IFNs, or of IFN with other antiviral or anticancer drugs, should also be more widely explored; there are already precedents to suggest that synergistic effects may be expected [*Fleischmann,* 1982]. Finally, we need to know more about the pharmacokinetics of the several IFNs; optimum dosage, routes and schedules have to be explored, and the in vivo stability of the molecule might be enhanced by genetic engineering or by developing novel modes of delivery.

J. Interferon Inducers

Shortly after the discovery of the induction of interferon by viruses, nonviral inducers of interferon were described. As discussed above, IFN-γ, once known as 'interferon II' or 'immune interferon', is induced by specific antigens which stimulate previously primed lymphocytes, or nonspecific mitogens which bind to unprimed lymphocytes [reviews: *Epstein,* 1981; *Vilček* et al., 1981]. On the other hand, IFN-α and -β may be produced by virtually any type of cell (including lymphocytes) following induction by viral or nonviral inducers. The latter include a wide variety of seemingly unrelated microorganisms, macromolecules, and lower molecular weight chemicals. The list is too long, and the data are too mixed in quality, to justify detailed attention in this review. For comprehensive treatment the reader is referred to the following books and reviews: *de Clercq* [1980]; *Stringfellow* [1980a, b]; *Torrence and de Clercq* [1977]; *Johnson and Baron* [1977]; *Pollard and Merigan* [1978].

Some general remarks are warranted, most of them conveying bad news. During the 1960s in particular, there was much interest in the development of substances capable of inducing interferon synthesis in man. At the time, interferon itself was prohibitively expensive and it seemed utterly logical to seek an inexpensive chemical that could convert the body into an interferon factory. Many and diverse types of natural and synthetic compounds, generally high-Mr polyanionic polymers [*Breinig and Morahan,* 1980; *Taylor and Grossberg,* 1982] were discovered to induce interferon, and sometimes to prevent, or even cure, viral infections in animals. Quite often, however, there was no demonstrable correlation between the induced interferon titer and the degree of protection against viral infection (or cancer). In all probability, the antiviral efficacy of many of these 'interferon inducers' has nothing whatever to do with interferon, but is a manifestation of some unrelated property, such as macrophage activation or immunomodulation [*Breinig and Morahan,* 1980; *Taylor and Grossberg,* 1982]. In other cases, compounds inducing good titers of interferon in a laboratory animal induced little or none in man; tilorone hydrochloride is a good example. Those that did were plagued by the problem of 'hyporesponsiveness' (hyporeactivity), discussed earlier, in which, following the first and subsequent doses of inducer, the individual becomes progressively more refractory to interferon induction. Furthermore, almost all of the inducers in the literature are too toxic for use in man. Indeed, none has yet been licensed for human administration. In the meantime, recombinant DNA technology has dramatically lowered the cost of production of interferon itself.

Nevertheless, work goes on, and some recent developments can be reported with guarded optimism. Following the original demonstration that dsRNA is the most effective inducer of interferon, a series of artificial dsRNAs, e.g., $(I)_n.(C)_n$, more widely known as polyI.polyC, were synthesized and demonstrated to be potent IFN inducers, but too toxic for use in man [review: *Gordon and Minks,* 1981]. However, in 1975 *Levy* and colleagues synthesized a complex of polyI.polyC with a polycation, poly-*L*-lysine; being insoluble, the complex was solubilized with carboxymethylcellose, hence the final product is known as poly(ICLC). Unlike polyI.polyC itself, poly(ICLC) is highly resistant to serum nucleases. It induced good titers of interferon in primates and man and protected primates against several lethal viruses, but was still somewhat toxic for man [*Levine* et al., 1979]. Then *Lampson* et al. [1982], simply by altering the ratio of polyI.polyC to poly-*L*-lysine in the complex, synthesized a 'polyI:C/poly-*L*-lysine' which was soluble, elicited high interferon titers in primates, and did not appear to lead to hyporesponsiveness following daily administration. Toxicity and protection studies in man have not been published to date.

Stringfellow [1980b] has addressed the problem of hyporesponsiveness in two ways. Working with a series of substituted 1,5-diamino-anthraquinones, which can be given orally (to mice), he presented evidence that hyporesponsiveness could be avoided by alternating different inducers. Secondly, he claimed that prostaglandins, administered with an inducer, can restore the response of hyporeactive animals.

V. Nucleoside Analogues

Most of the successful antiviral agents described to date (fig. 2) are nucleoside analogues, most of which in turn are restricted in their antiviral activity to the herpesviruses, especially herpes simplex and zoster [reviews: *Came and Caliguiri,* 1982; *Collier and Oxford,* 1980; *de Clercq,* 1981, 1982a; *Hahn,* 1980; *Walker* et al., 1979]. The prototype, 5-iodo-2′-deoxyuridine (IDU), was described by *Herrmann* [1961] and shown by *Kaufman* [1962] to be effective topically against HSV-1 infections of the eye. Trifluorothymidine (TFT) and adenine arabinoside (ara-A) followed. Then, in the late 1970s came what *de Clercq* [1981] describes as the 'second generation' of nucleoside analogues, most of which are much more selective by virtue of the fact that they require a virus-specific deoxythymidine-deoxycytidine kinase to phosphorylate them to the mono- or diphosphate; moreover, many of them (as the triphosphate) inhibit the viral DNA polymerase more efficiently than cellular DNA polymerase [reviews: *Elion,* 1980; *de Clercq* et al., 1980b, c; *de Clercq,* 1981, 1982a–c]. Hence, two distinct virus-coded enzymes are generally involved: one as activator of the antiviral agent, the other as its target. This second generation of nucleoside analogues includes, among many others:

Acyclovir	=	acycloguanosine
BVDU	=	(*E*)-5-(2-bromovinyl)-2′-deoxyuridine
FIAC	=	2′-fluoro-5-iodo-aracytosine
AIDDU	=	5′-amino-5-iodo-2′,5′-dideoxyuridine
ara-T	=	1-β-*D*-arabinofuranosyl thymine
DHPA	=	(S)-9-(2,3-dihydroxypropyl) adenine
Ribavirin	=	1-β-*D*-ribofuranosyl-1,2,4-triazole-3-carboxamide

The mode of action of some of the most active analogues is set out schematically in figure 3. Ribavirin and DHPA act quite differently from the others (and from one another, see below), which may account for their broader spectrum of activity against some families other than herpesviruses.

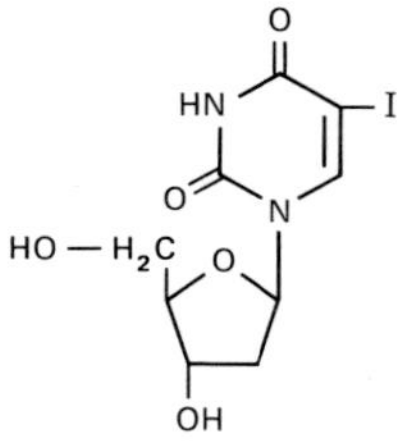

Idoxuridine (IDU)

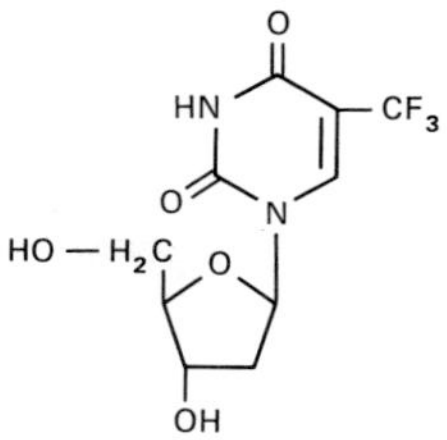

Trifluorothymidine (TFT)

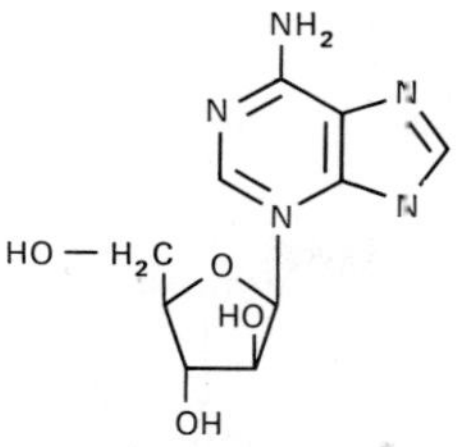

Adenine arabinoside (Ara-A)

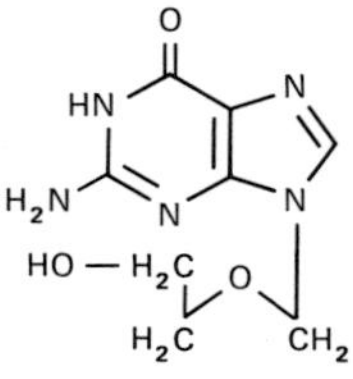

Acycloguanosine (Acyclovir)

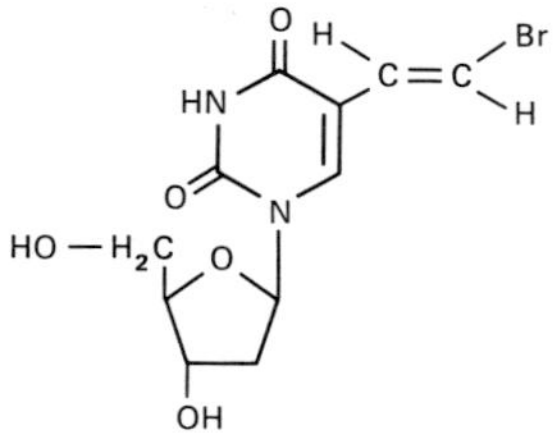

Bromovinyldeoxyuridine (BVDU)

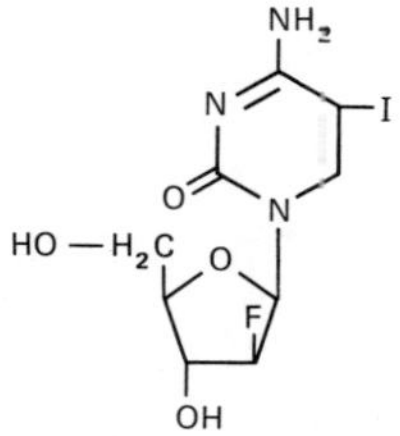

Fluoroiodoaracytosine (FIAC)

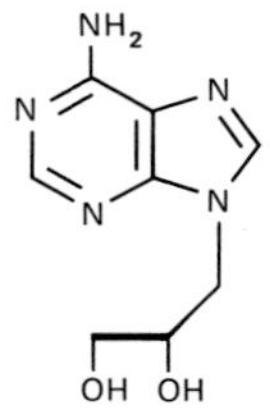

(S)-9-(2,3-Dihydroxypropyl) adenine (DHPA)

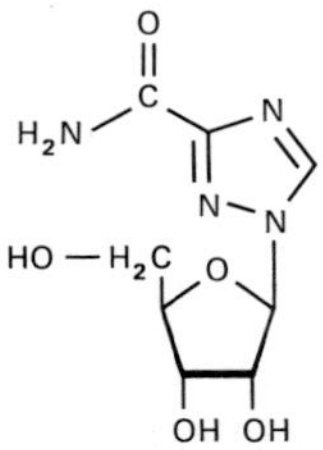

Ribavirin

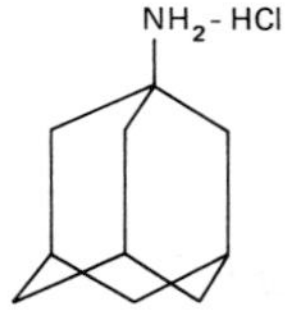

1-Adamantanamine hydrochloride (Amantadine)

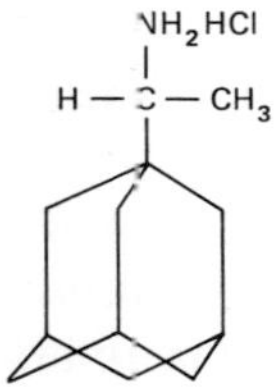

Rimantadine

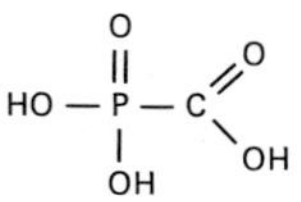

Phosphonoformic acid (PFA)

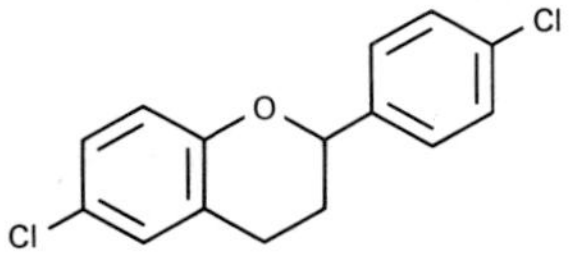

4',6-Dichloroflavan

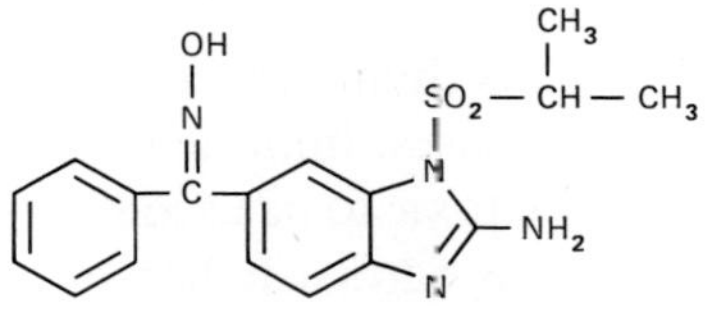

2-Amino-1-(isopropyl sulfonyl)-6-benzimidazole phenyl ketone oxime (Enviroxime)

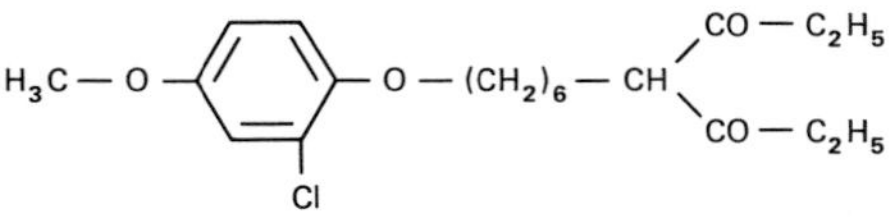

4-[6-(2-Chloro-4-methoxy) phenoxy] hexyl-3, 5-heptanedione (Arildone)

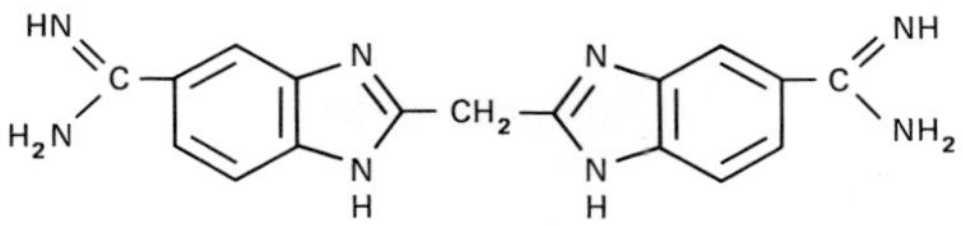

bis (5-Amidino-2-benzimidazolyl) methane

Fig. 2. Antiviral chemotherapeutic agents.

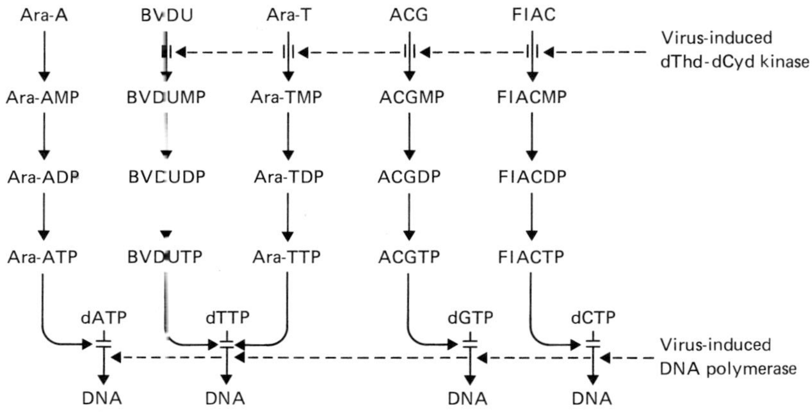

Fig. 3. Mechanism of inhibition of herpesvirus multiplication by nucleoside analogues. Reproduced in modified form from *de Clercq* [1981].

A. Idoxuridine (IDU)

Historically, 5-iodo-2′-deoxyuridine merits an honorable mention as the first antiviral chemotherapeutic agent to be licensed for human use [*Herrmann,* 1961; *Kaufman,* 1962] and the prototype of a long series of nucleoside analogues which were to prove effective against herpesviruses [reviews: *Bauer,* 1980a; *Oxford,* 1977; *Whitley and Alford,* 1981; *de Clercq,* 1982c].

This thymidine analogue, following phosphorylation in vivo by cellular kinases, inhibited both viral and cellular DNA synthesis. Hence it was too toxic to be used systemically but could be safely applied topically, as 0.1% eyedrops, to herpes simplex virus (HSV) infections localized to the eye. It has now been overtaken by the second-generation nucleoside analogues.

B. Trifluorothymidine (TFT)

Another halogenated nucleoside, trifluorothymidine, otherwise known as trifluridine, TFT or F_3T (fig. 2), largely superseded IDU for the treatment of HSV keratitis in the 1970s [*Wellings* et al., 1972]. Following phosphorylation by cellular kinases, TFT is thought to inhibit the enzyme thymidylate synthetase, thereby shutting off the production of dTTP without discrimination between viral and cellular DNA synthesis [*de Clercq,* 1982a]. Applied topically as 1% eye drops, F_3T is superior to both IDU and ara-A, and less commonly generates resistant mutants, but will probably in turn be replaced by acyclovir and BVDU (see below). The apparent synergism with interferon was mentioned earlier.

C. Adenine Arabinoside (Ara-A) and Ara-AMP

The first agent to be licensed for the treatment of systemic herpesvirus infections in man was adenine arabinoside, familiarly known as ara-A or Vidarabine [reviews: *Pavan-Langston* et al., 1975; *Whitley and Alford,* 1978, 1981; *Müller,* 1979; *North and Cohen,* 1979; *Buchanan and Hess,* 1980]. Ara-A or, to give it its full name, 9-β-*D*-arabinofuranosyladenine (fig. 2), was found to inhibit the replication of the human herpesviruses, HSV-1 and -2, varicella-zoster virus (VZV) and cytomegalovirus in cultured cells with a considerably better therapeutic index than idoxuridine. Like IDU, ara-A is phosphorylated by cellular enzymes, via ara-AMP and ara-ADP to ara-ATP, which blocks DNA synthesis by competitive inhibition of DNA polymerase and probably also by chain termination following incorporation into newly synthesized DNA strands [*Müller,* 1979; *North and Cohen,* 1979]. However, it is still not certain which, if any, of these effects accounts for its antiviral specificity; *de Clercq* [1982a] considers it unlikely to be the latter and points out that ara-A also inhibits S-adenosyl homocysteine hydrolase, ribonucleotide reductase, and polyadenylation of mRNA.

Ara-A is rapidly deaminated in vivo to form 9-β-*D*-arabinofuranosylhypoxanthine (ara-Hx), which displays much reduced antiviral activity. The in vivo efficacy (and toxicity) of ara-A can therefore be augmented up to 20-fold by competitive inhibitors of adenosine deaminase such as erythro-9-(2-hydroxy-3-nonyl) adenine (EHNA) [*North and Cohen,* 1979]. This could be useful clinically by allowing a reduction in the dose of ara-A. Ara-A is relatively insoluble, hence must be administered in a large volume of fluid by slow intravenous (i.v.) infusion. The usual dosage is (5–) 15 mg/kg/day in about (1–) 2 liters of fluid delivered i.v. over a 12-hour period each day for (5–) 10 days [*Whitley* et al., 1981; *Whitley and Alford,* 1981; *Galasso,* 1981a, b]. Particular caution must therefore be exercised in patients with kidney or liver dysfunction, and cerebral edema is a distinct risk. Manifestations of neurotoxicity are frequently reported. Furthermore, as might be expected with a drug that inhibits cellular DNA synthesis, toxic side effects referable to the gastrointestinal tract and bone marrow are not uncommon, particularly nausea, vomiting, diarrhea, thrombocytopenia, and leukopenia.

Clinically, ara-A has proven to be moderately effective in the early treatment of systemic herpes simplex viral infections. In a major controlled study, mortality in brain biopsy-proven HSV encephalitis was reduced from about 70 to 39%, though half the survivors displayed permanent sequelae; little or no therapeutic effect was demonstrable in older patients or patients already comatose before ara-A was commenced [*Whitley* et al., 1981]. In a recent trial of ara-A (15 mg/kg/day for 10 days by slow drip i.v. infusion) in neonatal (HSV-2) herpes, mortality was reduced from 86 to 57% in cases of disseminated disease and from 50 to 10% in localized CNS disease; in the localized mucocutaneous form of neonatal herpes, which is not fatal, the incidence of severe sequelae was reduced from 38% to zero [*Whitley and Alford,* 1981; *Galasso,* 1981a, b]. However, ara-A has no demonstrable effect on mucocutaneous HSV when applied topically to the skin. It is effective, as a 3% ophthalmic ointment, against HSV keratitis [*Buchanan and Hess,* 1980]. Herpes zoster and varicella in the immunocompromised also respond to i.v. ara-A [*Whitley and Alford,* 1981]. Zoster treated vigorously within 3 days of its first appearance responded with accelerated cutaneous healing, decreased dissemination and shortening of post-herpetic neuralgia [*Whitley* et al., 1982]. Most studies suggest that cytomegalovirus infections are refractory, although *Pollard* et al. [1980] presented results of an uncontrolled trial suggesting that CMV retinitis in immunosuppressed patients may respond to high doses of i.v. ara-A. *Scullard* et al. [1981] reported synergism between ara-A and interferon in the treatment of chronic active hepatitis B.

Adenine arabinoside monophosphate (ara-AMP) is much more soluble than ara-A, hence does not need to be delivered in large volumes of fluid, but can be administered intramuscularly or intravenously (25 mg/kg/day in 3 or 4 equal doses) [*Whitley and Alford,* 1981]. It has the additional advantage of being not subject to deamination by adenosine deaminase [*North and Cohen,* 1979]. Recent clinical trials indicate ara-AMP to be effective parenterally against HSV encephalitis, cutaneous herpes simplex and zoster in the immunosuppressed, but not topically against mucocutaneous or genital herpes simplex [*Whitley* et al., 1981; *Whitley and Alford,* 1981]. It was also effective against hepatitis B, especially when used in alternation with interferon.

D. Acycloguanosine (Acyclovir) and Homologues

A major breakthrough in antiviral chemotherapy occurred in 1977 when *Elion* and her colleagues [*Schaeffer* et al., 1978; *Elion* et al., 1977] developed an agent that depends upon a viral enzyme to convert it to its active form. Acycloguanosine, now commonly known as acyclovir or aciclovir, is a guanine derivative with an acyclic side chain, the full chemical name being 9-(2-hydroxyethoxymethyl) guanine (fig. 2) [reviews: *Bauer,* 1980a, b; *Elion,* 1980; *Brigden* et al., 1980, 1981; *King and Galasso,* 1982; *Field and Phillips,* 1983]. Its unique advantage over earlier nucleoside derivatives is that it requires the herpesvirus-specified enzyme, deoxythymidine-deoxycytidine (dThd-dCyd) kinase [*de Clercq,* 1982c] to phosphorylate it intracellularly to acycloguanosine monophosphate (acyclo GMP); a cellular GMP kinase then completes the phosphorylation to the active agent, acycloguanosine triphosphate (acyclo GTP). Acylo GTP inhibits the herpesvirus-specified DNA polymerase 10–30 times more effectively than it does cellular DNA polymerase; it acts as both inhibitor and substrate of the viral enzyme, competing with GTP and being incorporated into DNA, leading to chain termination because acyclovir lacks the 3′-hydroxyl group required for chain elongation [*Elion* et al., 1977; *Elion,* 1980]. Consequently, acyclovir is essentially nontoxic to uninfected cells but is powerfully inhibitory to viral DNA synthesis in infected cells.

Herpes simplex viruses types 1 and 2 are both very susceptible to acyclovir in cell culture; VZV is susceptible at somewhat higher concentrations of the drug [*Elion* et al., 1977; *Schaeffer* et al., 1978]. The other human herpesviruses, EB virus and cytomegalovirus, neither of which is known to possess a gene coding for thymidine kinase (TK), are nevertheless susceptible to acyclovir, albeit only at very much greater doses. In the case of EB virus this has been attributed to a particularly high sensitivity of the viral DNA polymerase to the small amount of acyclo GTP produced via the action of cellular enzymes [*Colby* et al., 1981]. Mouse cytomegalovirus, which also induces no TK, has been shown to be very sensitive to acyclovir, even in a TK^- strain of mouse 3T3 cells, suggesting that in this system acyclovir either does not require phosphorylation or is phosphorylated by a viral or cellular enzyme other than TK [*Burns* et al., 1981]. Recently, *de Clercq* [1982c] has pointed out that the so-called thymidine kinase induced by HSV and VZV is in fact a dThd-dCyd kinase, which recognizes both deoxythymidine and deoxycytidine as substrates; acyclovir is postulated to be perceived by the enzyme as a dCyd analogue, hence is phosphorylated not by dThd kinase but by dCyd kinase, for herpesviruses that induce a dThd kinase devoid of dCyd kinase activity are resistant to the drug. The relative sensitivity of different viruses seems to depend on a rather complex interplay of at least three variables : the efficiency of the virus-coded dThd-dCyd kinase (if any) in converting acyclovir to acyclo GMP; the efficiency of cellular kinases in converting this intermediate to acyclo GTP; and the susceptibility of the viral DNA polymerase to acyclo GTP.

In man, acyclovir displays marked activity against herpes simplex and varicella-zoster [*Selby* et al., 1979; reviews: *King and Galasso,* 1982; *Field and Phillips,* 1983]. Applied topically to the eye, acyclovir was first shown to be very effective against herpes simplex keratitis and corneal ulcers, being clearly superior to iododeoxyuridine [*Jones* et al., 1979] and at least as effective as TFT or ara-A [*King and Galasso,* 1982]. A double-blind, placebo-controlled trial of intravenous acyclovir in bone-marrow transplant recipients, who regularly suffer a reactivation of their latent herpes simplex in the 2nd week after transplantation, demonstrated 100% protection during the 18 days of prophylaxis, which commenced 3 days before the transplant [*Saral* et al., 1981]. Treatment of established mucocutaneous herpes simplex in patients immunosuppressed for the purpose of heart transplantation [*Chou* et al., 1981] or for a variety of other types of allograft or cancer [*Mitchell* et al., 1981] resulted in significant reductions in new lesions, symptoms and virus shedding.

Furthermore, acyclovir (ACV) is the first drug to offer some hope to herpes genitalis sufferers. Whether delivered topically [*Corey* et al., 1982], orally [*Nilsen* et al., 1982], or intravenously [*Mindel* et al., 1982], ACV reduces the duration of virus shedding, local pain/itching, and lesion-healing time, in primary herpes genitalis, though less persuasively in the (more short-lived) recurrent attacks [*King and Galasso,* 1982; *Field and Phillips,* 1983]. Unfortunately, there appears to be no significant reduction in the establishment of latency or in the frequency of subsequent recurrences. Oral treatment is of course the most convenient and evidently the most effective [*Nilsen* et al., 1982]. As no new lesions develop after the commencement of therapy, there is some prospect that the drug may prove to be more effective if administered promptly at the first indication of prodromal symptoms, which are experienced by about 2 out of every 3 patients. Self-medication with oral acyclovir has been shown to shorten the severity and duration of the disease and reduce virus shedding [*Bryson,* 1983]. Topical cream may have a place in self-management of relatively mild recurrences but is less effective than systemic treatment in reducing the incidence of urethritis and cervicitis, or virus shedding [*Corey* et al., 1983]. Intravenous therapy is probably only practicable for particularly severe primary infections requiring hospitalization. In the absence of any way of curing the latent state itself, the most attractive solution for herpes genitalis sufferers would undoubtedly be prevention of recurrences by long-term chemoprophylaxis. Preliminary trials along these lines have been very encouraging. Oral acyclovir, 200 mg 2–4 times daily, greatly reduced the frequency of attacks [see abstracts by *Douglas* et al., *Halsos* et al., *Kinghorn* et al. for 5th Int. Meeting Int. Soc. Sexually Transmitted Disease Research, 1983; and *Straus* et al., 1983]. Although no significant side effects were observed during trials lasting up to 4 months, careful longer-term studies will be necessary before prolonged chemoprophylaxis could be recommended as a routine.

So far, the results with herpes labialis (recurrent 'fever blisters' or 'cold sores') have not been quite so encouraging. Topical application of 5% acyclovir ointment (in polyethylene glycol) diminished virus shedding but had no benefical clinical effect [*Spruance* et al., 1982]. However, 5% acyclovir cream (in propylene glycol) did shorten healing time when applied 5 times per day for 5 days, especially if treatment was commenced before vesicles appeared [*Fiddian* et al., 1983]. Effective topical treatment of this common condition might require early application of cream to the area where lesions are known to recur, at the first indication of prodromal paresthesia.

Clinical trials in HSV encephalitis and neonatal herpes are in progress. The possibility also exists of protecting the infant by suppressing genital herpes by administering acyclovir to the mother prior to parturition, as an alternative to cesarean delivery.

Herpes zoster also responds well to ACV, at least following intravenous administration [*Peterslund* et al., 1979; *Selby* et al., 1979; *King and Galasso,* 1982]; no new lesions develop, and pain is reduced but often returns on withdrawal of therapy. In immunocompromised patients with varicella-zoster infections, intravenous acyclovir reduced the incidence of progression to visceral varicella or zoster [*Balfour* et al., 1983]. Unfortunately, however, there was no significant effect, in normal or immunocompromised persons, on that most distressing sequela, post-herpetic neuralgia. In view of the ineffectiveness (against zoster) of oral acyclovir at the usual dosage of 1 g daily, trials have been initiated using considerably higher dosage. ACV has been disappointing against other herpesviruses.

Most studies have revealed no effect against cytomegalovirus (congenital CMID of infants, or CMV pneumonia following bone marrow transplantation), nor against EB virus [*Field and Phillips,* 1983].

Acyclovir (Zovirax) may be delivered by slow intravenous infusion over at least a 1-hour period (5–10 mg/kg every 8 h for at least 5 days), or orally (e.g., 200 mg 5 times daily for 5–10 days), or topically. As anticipated from in vitro studies, the drug seems to be nontoxic. Rapid transient increases in blood urea and creatinine levels tend to occur [*Selby* et al., 1979], particularly if the drug is given as a bolus i.v. injection. Intramuscular injection is painful, and severe local inflammatory reactions follow accidental subcutaneous injection. Acyclovir levels must be carefully monitored in patients with dehydration or renal impairment, as the drug, which is excreted unchanged through the kidneys, is rather insoluble, and crystalluria may occur [*Brigden* et al., 1980]. Elevated liver enzymes have been reported in immunocompromised subjects. Ophthalmic ointment (3% acyclovir) stings some patients, and reversible punctate keratopathy is commonly observed. Ointments originally developed for application to skin and mucous membranes contain 5% acyclovir in a polyethylene glycol base. However, recent trials indicate the superiority of an aqueous cream containing 5% acyclovir in propylene glycol [*Fiddian* et al., 1983].

Acyclovir-resistant mutants of herpes simplex virus readily develop in cell culture. The mutations can be located in either the gene coding for the viral thymidine kinase (TK) or that for DNA polymerase [*Coen and Schaffer,* 1980; *Schnipper and Crumpacker,* 1980; *Field* et al., 1981; *Furman* et al., 1981]. There appear to be two kinds of TK^- mutant: those failing to induce appreciable levels of TK, and those in which the enzyme is produced in good amounts but has an altered substrate specificity such that it can no longer satisfactorily phosphorylate acyclovir [*Darby* et al., 1981]. The DNA polymerase mutants may also be of more than one kind; while all are assumed to have reduced sensitivity to acyclo GTP [*Crumpacker* et al., 1982], only some of them display cross-resistance to phosphonoacetic acid [*Furman* et al., 1981]. None of the mutants yet described shows cross-resistance against F_3T or ara-A, but TK^- mutants are resistant to bromovinyldeoxyuridine (BVDU, see below) as well as to acyclovir, because both agents require phosphorylation by this viral enzyme [*Field* et al., 1981]. Acyclovir-resistant mutants of the TK^- class have been isolated from man following acyclovir therapy [*Burns* et al., 1982] and demonstrated to be resistant also to BVDU [*Crumpacker* et al., 1982]. It has been suggested that such TK^- mutants will not pose a serious threat because, in mice at least, they tend to display reduced pathogenicity [*Field and Wildy,* 1978] and reduced capacity to establish latent infection in the trigeminal ganglion [*Tenser* et al., 1979].

Recently, derivatives of acyclovir, such as 9-{[2-hydroxy-1-(hydroxymethyl)ethoxy]methyl}guanine, otherwise known as 2′-nor-2′-deoxyguanosine (2′-NDG), or BIOLF-62, have been shown to be even more efficient substrates for HSV-1 thymidine kinase and GMP kinase than is acyclovir itself, and display greater activity against herpes simplex virus in cultured cells and mice [*Smith* et al., 1982; *Ashton* et al., 1982]. Clinical investigations have begun on a number of such analogues, including some that are better absorbed than acyclovir following oral delivery, and are then converted to acyclovir, giving higher serum levels.

E. Bromovinyldeoxyuridine (BVDU) and Homologues

Following the example set by acycloguanosine, a wide range of other nucleoside analogues with similar modes of action have now been synthesized [reviews: *de Clercq* et al., 1980b, c; *de Clercq,* 1982c]. Of these, one of the most promising is *(E)*-5-(2-bromovinyl)-2′-deoxyuridine (BVDU) (fig. 2), developed in Belgium by *de Clercq* et al. [1979] [review: *de Clercq,* 1982b]. BVDU is a nontoxic anti-herpetic agent which requires the virus-induced deoxythymidine (dThd) kinase to convert it to BVDU monophosphate (BVDUMP). Unlike acyclovir, BVDU is effective against a variety of nonhuman herpesviruses which induce dThd kinase without a dCyd kinase activity, hence it is believed that deoxythymidine kinase is indeed the enzyme that phosphorylates the drug [*de Clercq,* 1982c]. The cellular kinases complete the phosphorylation to BVDU triphosphate (BVDUTP), which is the active form of the agent. The viral DNA polymerase is considerably more susceptible to BVDUTP than are the cellular DNA polymerases α, β and γ.

HSV-1 virus multiplication is inhibited by BVDU at concentrations down to 0.01 μg/ml, i.e., about 5–10 times lower than the minimum effective concentration of acyclovir, and 3,000–10,000 times lower than the BVDU dose inhibiting cellular DNA synthesis [*de Clercq* et al., 1980b; *de Clercq,* 1982b]. As expected, the drug is virtually ineffective against TK^- mutants of HSV-1. HSV-2 is 150–200 times less sensitive than HSV-1; this may be explained by the finding that the HSV-2 dThd kinase phosphorylates BVDU only to its monophosphate, whereas HSV-1 kinase converts the drug to the diphosphate. Varicella-zoster virus (VZV) is even more sensitive than HSV-1 to BVDU, the 50% inhibitory concentration being 0.001–0.01 μg/ml [*Machida* et al., 1982], hence it seems likely that BVDU will turn out to be considerably more effective against this virus in vivo than acyclovir. Even more striking selectivity for VZV has been achieved with a BVDU derivative, [1-β-*D*-arabinofuranosyl-(*E*)-5-(2-bromovinyl)uracil], known as BVaraU, which inhibits the multiplication of VZV in cell culture at a minimum concentration of 1 ng/ml [*de Clercq,* 1982b; *Machida* et al., 1982].

BVDU is very effective by mouth (5–15 mg/kg/day for 5 days), and this route of administration appears to be quite satisfactory for the treatment of systemic herpesvirus infections. Uncontrolled clinical trials against mucocutaneous HSV [*de Clercq* et al., 1980b] and varicella-zoster [*de Clercq* et al., 1980a] in cancer patients look very promising indeed. During only 5 days' treatment existing lesions rapidly regressed and no new lesions appeared [*de Clercq,* 1982b]. Furthermore, no toxic side effects were detected. As with acyclovir, BVDU is somewhat impeded by the blood-brain barrier, which may limit its effectiveness against HSV encephalitis. It is very effective as 0.1% eyedrops in the treatment of HSV keratitis and dendritic corneal ulcers [*de Clercq* et al., 1980b; *de Clercq,* 1982b]. The results of double-blind, placebo-controlled trials of BVDU against the whole range of herpesvirus infections are eagerly awaited.

Recently, *de Clercq* et al. [1982] have reported that 5-substituted 2'-deoxycytidines are more selective in their anti-HSV activity than the corresponding 5-substituted 2'-deoxyuridines, presumably because of the requirement that, following the phosphorylation of the drug by the HSV-coded enzyme, dThd-dCyd kinase, the dCMP analogue must then be deaminated to the corresponding dUMP analogue by a second (virus-coded?) enzyme, dCMP deaminase. Accordingly, 5-X-dCyd derivatives are less cytotoxic than their dUrd counterparts. Bromovinyldeoxycytidine and iodovinyldeoxycytidine were the most potent and selective of this series as inhibitors of HSV in cell culture.

F. Fluoroiodoaracytosine (FIAC)

Watanabe et al. [1979] described a new agent, 2'-fluoro-5-iodo-1-β-*D*-arabinofuranosylcytosine (FIAC) (fig. 2), which also requires phosphorylation by the virus-induced enzyme, dThd-dCyd kinase [*de Clercq,*

1982c]. It is very potent and displays a high chemotherapeutic index against HSV (types 1 and 2), VZV and some strains of cytomegalovirus in cultured cells [see also *de Clercq* et al., 1980c]. Clinical trials indicate efficacy of intravenous FIAC against herpes simplex and zoster. A related compound, 2′-fluoro-5-methyl-ara-U, known as FMAU, was more effective than FIAC against HSV-1 in mice.

G. S-Adenosyl-Homocysteine Analogues

3-Deazaadenosine and (*S*)-9-(2,3-dihydroxypropyl) adenine (DHPA) (fig. 2) are two of several compounds that have been shown to inhibit the cellular enzyme, SAH hydrolase, leading to the accumulation of S-adenosylhomocysteine (SAH), which inhibits methyltransfer from the methyl donor SAM (S-adenosylmethionine) to the 5′-cap of messenger RNA [*Bader* et al., 1978; *de Clercq,* 1982a]. It is not yet clear whether methylation of viral mRNA is inhibited preferentially, but DHPA has been reported to have some effect against rabies and rotavirus in animal models [*de Clercq,* 1982a].

H. Ribavirin (Virazole)

A rather different nucleoside analogue, known as ribavirin or Virazole [reviews: *Sidwell* et al., 1979; *Smith and Kirkpatrick,* 1980] was first synthesized in 1972 but, despite extensive investigation, has still not been licensed for use in many countries, partly because of unpersuasive evidence of antiviral activity in man and partly because of indications of toxicity. Superficially, the drug would appear to have considerable potential, as it inhibits the growth of a wide spectrum of RNA and DNA viruses in cultured cells and experimental animals. However, this early promise has not so far been matched by a comparable degree of efficacy in humans.

Ribavirin or, to give it its full name, 1-β-*D*-ribofuranosyl-1,2,4-triazole-3-carboxamide (fig. 2), is structurally related to guanosine, which can reverse its effect. Cellular adenosine kinase phosphorylates ribavirin intracellularly to its 5′-monophosphate, which in turn competitively inhibits IMP dehydrogenase, an enzyme involved in guanosine monophosphate biosynthesis. This would suggest that ribavirin monophosphate may exert its antiviral (and, to a more limited extent, anticellular) effects by reducing intracellular guanosine nucleotide pools. But ribavirin exists intracellularly mainly as ribavirin-5′-triphosphate, and this has been shown to inhibit the enzyme, mRNA guanylyltransferase, responsible for addition of the 7-methylguanosine 'cap' to the 5′-terminus of viral mRNA [*Smith and Kirkpatrick,* 1980]. This is consistent with the drug's broad spectrum of activity against both RNA viruses of negative polarity and DNA viruses, but casts doubt on the selectivity of the agent, for cellular mRNA is also capped. The sensitivity of influenza virus might reflect the peculiar requirement of that virus that the 5′-cap (and adjacent nucleotides) be transferred from cellular mRNA to viral mRNA [*Plotch* et al., 1979]. It has also been claimed that ribavirin triphosphate inhibits influenza viral RNA polymerase directly [*Eriksson* et al., 1977].

It is not yet clear why ribavirin inhibits some viruses but not others in cell culture, nor why in vivo experience does not regularly bear out in vitro indications. Perhaps the most encouraging results in vivo so far have been with the highly dangerous arenaviruses, Lassa and Machupo, and the bunyavirus of Rift Valley fever [*Smith and Kirkpatrick,* 1980]. Very high doses of the drug, given systemically, protected monkeys against the lethal effects of Lassa fever [*Jahrling* et al., 1980]. Earlier claims of efficacy for oral ribavirin against influenza in man have not been substantiated, although *Knight* et al. [1980, 1981] reported good results when the drug was administered for prolonged periods as an aerosol through a respirator. *Hall* et al. [1983] have recently reported similar success in the treatment of infants hospitalized with lower respiratory infections attributable to respiratory syncytial virus; continuous exposure to an aerosol of ribavirin in the tent in which the babies were held for 3–6 days reduced the severity and duration of the illness and the titer of virus in the lungs. Reports of activity against hepatitis viruses and herpesviruses [*Smith and Kirkpatrick,* 1980] await confirmation.

There are some grounds for concern that the use of ribavirin for non-life-threatening diseases such as influenza or cutaneous herpesvirus infections of healthy people may not be justified because of its toxic side effects. Following oral administration at the usual dosage of about 1 g per day, a substantial minority (up to 25%) of recipients develop a reversible anemia with increased reticulocyte numbers and elevated serum bilirubin levels; moreover, the immunosuppressive and teratogenic potential of the drug demonstrable in animals [*Powers* et al., 1982] requires more detailed study [*Oxford,* 1977; *Galasso* et al., 1979; *Sidwell* et al., 1979; *Smith and Kirkpatrick,* 1980].

VI. Other Antiviral Agents

A. Methisazone

Methisazone, or N-methylisatin β-thiosemicarbazone, enjoys the double distinction of being the first true antiviral chemotherapeutic agent to be described and the only one to be rendered redundant by the eradication of the virus against which it was directed, namely smallpox. The biochemistry and pharmacology of the agent, which have been quite intensively studied, were reviewed by *Bauer* [1977].

B. Trisodium Phosphonoformate (PFA)

In 1973 an anti-herpetic agent known as phosphonoacetate was first described [review: *Boezi,* 1979]. This simple compound, which binds directly to the pyrophosphate binding site of the viral DNA polymerase, is active in vivo, but is extremely irritating to skin when applied topically and is retained by bone whatever the route of administration, hence is unlikely to be licensed for human use.

However, in 1978, a related compound, trisodium phosphonoformate, known also as phosphonoformic acid (PFA, or foscarnet) (fig. 2) was found to inhibit the DNA polymerase of the herpesviruses, HSV-1 and human cytomegalovirus, at 10–100 times lower concentration than required to inhibit cellular DNA polymerase α; there is also a discernible but much less selective affinity for the DNA polymerase of hepatitis B virus and the reverse transcriptase of retrovirus [review: *Helgstrand* et al., 1980]. Mutants with a PFA-resistant DNA polymerase have been obtained.

Clinical trials in man so far indicate that 3% PFA cream, which is not irritating to skin, shortens the time mucocutaneous herpes simplex type 1 or 2 lesions take to reach the stage of crusting and reduces the appearance of new vesicles [*Helgstrand* et al., 1980]. Topical treatment of recurrent genital herpes with foscarnet cream has also been claimed to accelerate healing, especially in men [*Wallin* et al., 1983].

Some 30% of systemically available PFA is deposited in bone and cartilage. Although toxicity for man has not yet been reported, this will need to be carefully checked, in the long term as well as the short, especially before PFA is licensed for oral or systemic administration.

C. Arildone

Arildone or, to give it its full name, 4-[6-(2-chloro-4-methoxy)phenoxyl]hexyl-3,5-heptanedione (fig. 2), represents a new class of antiviral chemotherapeutic agents (aryloxyl alkyl diketones) which display some selectivity against a number of RNA and DNA viruses in cell culture [*Diana* et al., 1977]. It has been shown to inhibit uncoating of the polio virion in cultured cells [*McSharry* et al., 1979] and to limit the multiplication of poliovirus in mice [*McKinlay* et al., 1982]. Arildone and its pyrazole derivative, 4-[6-(2-chloro-4-methoxyphenoxy)hexyl]-3,5-diethyl-1-H-pyrazole methane sulfonate [*Pancic* et al., 1981] in dimethyl sulfoxide (DMSO) are active topically against HSV-1 and HSV-2 infections in laboratory animals and are currently undergoing clinical trials in man.

D. Amantadine and Rimantadine

It is now some 20 years since a simple three-ringed symmetrical amine, known as 1-aminoadamantane hydrochloride or, more commonly, as amantadine (fig. 2), was synthesized and shown to inhibit the replication of influenza A viruses [*Davies* et al., 1964]. The mode of action of the drug is still not completely understood. Earlier claims that it inhibits penetration or uncoating of the virion are now disputed [review: *Oxford and Galbraith,* 1980], but *Helenius* et al. [1980] have postulated that amantadine does indeed block uncoating by increasing the pH in the lysosome and so preventing the pH 5 mediated fusion with the viral envelope. *Skehel* et al. [1978] presented evidence that the block occurs after uncoating, primary transcription of RNA being inhibited. Amantadine resistance, which develops quite readily, is often associated with the gene coding for the M protein [*Lubeck* et al., 1978; *Hay* et al., 1979], but this is not invariably so [*Scholtissek and Faulkner,* 1979].

Amantadine, administered orally, inhibits the multiplication of influenza A viruses of all subtypes (H1, H2, H3) but, strangely, not influenza B or C [review: *Couch and Jackson,* 1976; *Oxford and Galbraith,* 1980; *Galasso,* 1981a, b]. Though its effectiveness has been questioned [*Sabin,* 1978], published clinical trials indicate a consensus that the drug can reduce the incidence of clinical influenza by up to 90% if administered prophylactically [*Dolin* et al., 1982]. In practice, this demands the ingestion of 200 mg daily for 6 weeks from the commencement of an influenza epidemic in the community. Therapeutically, the agent is much less effective, but has been reported to reduce the severity of symptoms.

Side effects commonly occur (7–33% of patients in various studies). They relate mainly to the central nervous system – loss of concentration, insomnia, nervousness, light-headedness, drowsiness, anxiety, confusion – but are generally reversible and mild unless the recommended dose is exceeded, or the patient has a history of mental illness or renal disease [*Couch and Jackson,* 1976; *Oxford,* 1977; *Galasso* et al., 1979; *Oxford and Galbraith,* 1980; *Collier and Oxford,* 1980; *Galasso,* 1981a, b].

Rimantadine, or α-methyl-1-adamantane-methylamine hydrochloride (fig. 2), found to be more active and less toxic in cultured cells, organ cultures and experimental animals, has been extensively used in the USSR for several years. Since side effects are less frequent and less severe than with amantadine and efficacy is comparable [*Couch and Jackson,* 1976; *Galasso* et al., 1979; *Dolin* et al., 1982], rimantadine is clearly the drug of choice.

Like amantadine, rimantadine is given orally, but there is some interest in the possibility of delivering either drug by aerosol spray, perhaps in conjunction with ribavirin [*Knight* et al., 1980, 1981].

E. Enviroxime and Benzimidazoles

Many years ago, *Tamm* and his colleagues described a group of benzimidazole derivatives which displayed in vitro, but not in vivo, activity against picornaviruses, attributed at the time to inhibition of initiation of viral RNA synthesis [*Caliguiri and Tamm,* 1973]. Subsequently, *Eggers* [1976] demonstrated that, despite relatively low therapeutic indices, 2-(α-hydroxybenzyl)-benzimidazole (HBB) and guanidine act synergistically to protect newborn mice from death following infection with enteroviruses. Then, in 1981 *Phillpotts* et al. reported that 2-amino-1-(isopropyl-sulfonyl)-6-benzimidazole phenyl ketone oxime (enviroxime) (fig. 2) was effective prophylactically in subsequent trials against rhinovirus type 9 in man, when delivered simultaneously by mouth and nasal spray. However, adverse side effects, principally nausea and vomiting, attributed to the oral enviroxime, were unacceptably frequent. Intranasal therapy alone proved ineffective, even prophylactically, against rhinovirus type 4 [*Levandowski* et al., 1982] or type 39 [*Hayden and Gwaltney,* 1982].

F. Flavans

A recently described flavan derivative, 4′-6-dichloroflavan (fig. 2), inhibits the replication of many (but not all) serotypes of rhinovirus in cell culture [*Bauer* et al., 1981]. Its mode of action is unclear but it binds (reversibly) to virions and seems to act shortly after entry of the virion into the cell [*Tisdale and Selway,* 1983]. Preliminary tests in animals indicate that it is absorbed from the gut and is nontoxic. Trials in man have so far been discouraging [*Phillpotts* et al., 1983].

A Japanese group has now described a series of related naturally occurring compounds displaying activity against picornaviruses. One of these, 4′-ethoxy-2′-hydroxy-4,6′-dimethoxychalcone (Ro 09-0410), inhibits the replication of most rhinoviruses (but not other picornaviruses) in HeLa cells at 0.03 μg/ml, with a therapeutic index of 10^3, apparently acting by binding directly to the virion itself [*Ishitsuka* et al., 1982].

VII. Other Possible Approaches

A. Virus-Specific Oligonucleotides

A short synthetic sequence of single-stranded DNA complementary to the 13 nucleotides of the 3′- and 5′-reiterated terminal sequences of Rous sarcoma virus RNA inhibits both virus production and cell transformation [*Zamecnik and Stephenson,* 1978]. On the other hand, an oligodeoxyribonucleotide complementary to the 12 nucleotides at the 3′-terminus of influenza viral (–) RNA failed to block transcription selectively [*Stridh* et al., 1981]. It remains to be seen whether this novel approach to antiviral chemotherapy has any general validity.

B. Virus-Specific Oligopeptides and Inhibitors of Proteases

Penetration of ortho- and paramyxoviruses by fusion requires prior cleavage of a viral envelope glycoprotein by a cellular protease. Hence, synthetic oligopeptides that mimic the amino acid sequence in the vicinity of the specific cleavage site might conceivably block viral multiplication. *Norrby* [1971] had shown that a particular tripeptide carrying a carbobenzoxy group (Z) on the N-terminal amino acid prevented the multiplication of measles virus by inhibiting its penetration into cells. Following up this observation, *Richardson* et al. [1980] demonstrated that oligopeptides with an amino acid sequence resembling the N-terminal sequence of the F_1 polypeptide which is exposed by cleavage of the paramyxovirus F (fusion) protein, or of the influenza HA_2 protein, specifically inhibit multiplication of the respective viruses in cell culture. Antiviral activity in vivo has yet to be demonstrated, however.

Korant [1981] has generalized this proposal and postulated that, since cleavage of viral proteins by proteases, some of which are virus-coded, is required at several stages in the multiplication cycle, including not only entry by fusion but also activation of some viral enzymes, post-translational cleavage of the 'polyprotein' product of polycistronic mRNA, and assembly of the virion, it should be possible to find or devise agents mimicking the cleavage site and thus specifically inhibiting the virus-coded protease.

Various diarylamidine derivatives inhibit trypsin-like proteases [*Tidwell* et al., 1978]. Some of these, such as bis(5-amidino-2-benzimidazolyl)-methane (fig. 2), prevent respiratory syncytial virus-induced cell fusion [*Dubovi* et al., 1981], but it has yet to be demonstrated that the observed inhibition of virus penetration is due to competition between the drug and the F glycoprotein for the putative protease. Yields of virus are not reduced significantly following intranasal administration of the drug to cotton rats.

C. Entry of Inhibitors through Permeable Membranes

Carrasco [1978, 1981] presented evidence that virus-infected cells become permeable to charged molecules of low Mr, early as well as later in infection, and suggested that this could form the basis for a novel approach to a antiviral chemotherapy, namely the use of low-Mr inhibitors, e.g., of protein synthesis or nucleic acid synthesis [*Gauri,* 1981], that are incapable of penetrating uninfected cells. However, it seems likely that the 'leaky membranes' he observes occur neither early enough nor reliably enough to be exploited successfully or safely in vivo.

D. Inhibitors of Glycosylation

The multiplication of viruses that bud from membranes is blocked by inhibitors of glycoprotein synthesis [*Gandhi* et al., 1972]. Such agents, of course, inhibit the synthesis of cellular glycoproteins as well, but it is possible that they might be safely applied topically to epithelial surfaces such as skin, eye or genital tract, and/or that agents might be developed which selectively block the addition of particular oligosaccharides more characteristic of given viruses than of the host cell [review: *Klenk and Schwarz,* 1982].

E. Inhibitors of Reverse Transcriptase

Diarylamidine derivatives seem to have a second, distinct antiviral activity, namely inhibition of reverse transcriptase. *Larnicol* et al. [1981] have reported that these and other inhibitors of this enzyme block the development of retrovirus-induced leukemia in mice. Quite a number of agents with various modes of action (including, for example, the anti-tuberculosis drug, rifampicin) are now known to inhibit reverse transcriptase [*de Clercq,* 1979, 1982a]; their relevance to medicine will depend not only on their selectivity for the viral enzyme but also upon whether retroviruses are responsible for a significant proportion of cancer in man.

VIII. Summary

Table V summarizes the modes of action of the major antiviral chemotherapeutic agents discussed in this review. Table VI indicates the viruses against which they have been shown unequivocally to be effective in man.

Table V. Mechanism of action of antiviral chemotherapeutic agents

Target	Drug	via
Entry		
Cleavage of envelope protein (protease)	diarylamidines	
	virus-specific oligopeptides	
Uncoating	arildone	
	amantadine, rimantadine	
Primary transcription	specific oligonucleotides	
RNA-dependent RNA polymerase	ribavirin →	RTP
Reverse transcriptase	diarylamidines	
Processing of mRNA		
3′-Polyadenylation	Ara-A, Ara-AMP →	Ara-ATP
5′-Capping (mRNA guanylyltransferase)	ribavirin →	RTP
5′-Capping (SAH hydrolase)	DHPA	
	Ara-A, Ara-AMP →	Ara-ATP
5′-Capping (AdoMet & AdoHcy)	interferons	

Table V (continued)

Target	Drug	via
Translation		
mRNA degradation by activation of endoribonuclease	interferons $\xrightarrow{\text{dsRNA}}$ activated 2-5A synthetase $\rightarrow$	2-5A → RNase L
Phosphorylation of initiation factor, eIF-2	interferons $\xrightarrow{\text{dsRNA}}$	activated protein kinase
Replication of viral DNA		
DNA polymerase	Ara-A, Ara-AMP →	Ara-ATP
	acyclovir $\xrightarrow{\text{viral dThd-dCyd kinase}}$	ACVTP
	BVDU $\xrightarrow{\text{viral dThd kinase}}$	BVDUTP
	FIAC $\xrightarrow{\text{viral dThd-dCyd kinase}}$	FIACTP
	phosphonoformic acid	
IMP dehydrogenase	ribavirin →	RMP
Adenosine deaminase	DHPA	
Thymidylate synthetase	trifluorothymidine →	TFTMP
Incorporation into DNA	idoxuridine →	IDUTP
	Ara-A, Ara-AMP →	Ara-ATP
	acylovir $\xrightarrow{\text{viral dThd-dCyd kinase}}$	ACVTP
	BVDU $\xrightarrow{\text{viral dThd kinase}}$	BVDUTP
	FIAC $\xrightarrow{\text{viral dThd-dCyd kinase}}$	FIACTP
Replication of vRNA	enviroxime	
Processing of viral protein		
Post-translational cleavage [protease(s)]	diarylamidines	

Table VI. Antiviral agents of proven efficacy in man

Agent	Virus
Interferon α, β, γ	hepatitis B, papilloma, herpesviruses, respiratory viruses, cancer?
Nucleoside Analogues	
Idoxuridine (IDU)	herpes simplex
Trifluorothymidine (TFT)	herpes simplex
Adenine arabinoside (ara-A) and Ara-AMP	herpes simplex; varicella-zoster; hepatitis B
Acycloguanosine (acyclovir)	herpes simplex; varicella-zoster
Bromovinyldeoxyuridine (BVDU)	herpes simplex; varicella-zoster
Ribavirin (Virazole)	influenza; respiratory syncytial virus
Other antiviral agents	
Trisodium phosphonoformate (PFA)	herpes simplex
Amantadine and rimantadine	influenza A

IX. Classification of Vaccines

Readers will no doubt be familiar with the distinction between live (attenuated) and inactivated vaccines. We shall do no more than tabulate the properties perceived as advantages and disadvantages of live versus inactivated vaccines (table VII); the arguments have been widely debated over many years and continue to be at issue today [*Sabin,* 1981b; *Salk,*

Table VII. Advantages and disadvantages of live versus dead vaccines

	Live	Inactivated
Route of administration	natural[a] or injection	injection
Dose of virus; cost	low	high
Number of doses	single[b]	multiple
Need for adjuvant	no	yes[c]
Duration of immunity	many years	generally less[d]
Antibody response	IgG; IgA[e]	IgG
Cell-mediated response	good	poor
Heat lability in tropics	yes[f]	no
Interference	occasional; OPV only[g]	no
Side effects	occasional mild symptoms[h]	no
Reversion to virulence	rarely; OPV only[i]	no

[a] Oral or respiratory, in certain cases.
[b] Except OPV (to preempt possibility of interference). For some other live vaccines a single booster may be required by law (yellow fever) or desirable (rubella?) after a decade or so.
[c] But few satisfactory adjuvants yet licensed for human use.
[d] But satisfactory with some inactivated vaccines.
[e] IgA if delivered via oral or respiratory route. OPV can thereby prevent wild poliovirus from multiplying in the gut, hence facilitate near-eradication of the virus from the community.
[f] $MgCl_2$ and other stabilizers, plus maintenance of 'cold chain' assist preservation.
[g] Especially in Third World.
[h] Especially rubella and measles.
[i] 10^{-6} vaccinees.

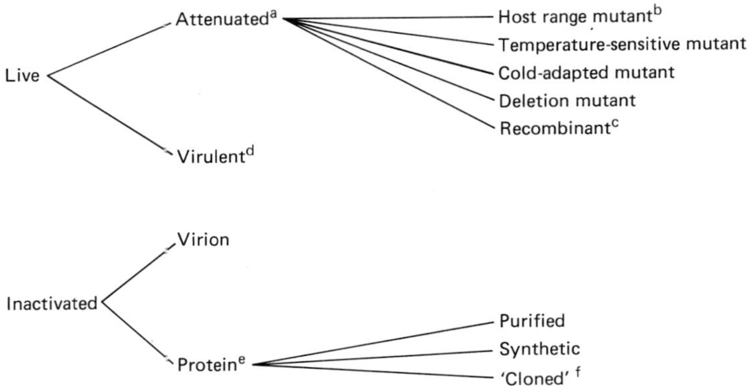

Fig. 4. Types of viral vaccine. (a) Including genetic reassortants incorporating mutant genes. (b) Occurring naturally in a different animal species, or selected by passage in cultured cells. (c) Incorporating gene from another virus. (d) Delivered via an unnatural route or at a safe age (in veterinary medicine). (e) May be incorporated in liposome or adjuvant. (f) In prokaryotic or eukaryotic cells by recombinant DNA technology.

1980; *Melnick,* 1978, 1980; *Chanock and Murphy,* 1980]. Immunological considerations, as well as those of safety and vaccination policy, are discussed at length elsewhere [*Mims and White,* 1984]. Suffice to add here that there is no absolute answer to this difficult dilemma. The theoretical virtues and limitations of the two contending approaches may be overshadowed in practice by the track record of particular vaccines in the field. Furthermore, the choice no longer lies between the two classical protagonists: the host range mutant and the inactivated whole virus. The large number of novel approaches to the derivation of vaccines introduced during the past few years (fig. 4) means that we can no longer generalize about 'live' and 'dead' vaccines in quite such a simplistic fashion. The merits and demerits of each new type of vaccine must be independently assessed.

X. New Approaches to Vaccine Design

A. Temperature-Sensitive and Cold-Adapted Mutants

The first major departure from the classical, largely empirical procedures for derivation of live viral vaccines by the selection of host-range mutants via serial passage in cell culture was attributable to *Chanock* and his associates at the US National Institutes of Health. Building on the notion put forward by *Fenner* [1972] that temperature-sensitive *(ts)* mutants presented a logical approach to viral vaccines, they devoted much of the 1970s to the development of *ts* vaccines against influenza and respiratory syncytial virus [reviews: *Chanock and Murphy,* 1980; *Chanock,* 1981; *Murphy and Chanock,* 1981]. As predicted, such vaccines, administered intranasally, were avirulent yet immunogenic. The bad news, however, was that even mutants containing multiple *ts* mutations tended to revert towards virulence in vivo with unacceptable frequency. Surprisingly, this was found not to be due to simple back-mutation but to suppressor mutations occurring in seemingly unrelated genes [*Murphy* et al., 1980]. This disappointment, coupled with concern voiced in some quarters about the theoretical possibility that *ts* mutants might display an enhanced propensity to establish persistent infections, perhaps in the brain [for discussion, see *Richman and Murphy,* 1979] led to the reluctant abandonment of this particular approach to vaccine design.

Not to be denied, however, *Murphy and Chanock* [1981] turned their attention to a somewhat different approach pioneered by *Maassab.* 'Cold-adapted' *(ca)* mutants grow optimally at a temperature lower than that of the body, say 25–33 °C, but not at 37 °C. Hence they multiply satisfactorily in the nose but should not be capable of spreading to involve the lungs or other vulnerable parts of the body. *Maassab* et al. [1981] have produced a master strain of influenza virus containing a mutation in every gene. Genetic reassortants constructed from six of these genes plus the HA and NA genes from the prevalent wild strain show little reversion in man [*Murphy and Chanock,* 1981; *Kendal* et al., 1982].

B. Deletion Mutants

In theory one might predict a negligible reversion rate in 'deletion mutants' lacking part of their nucleic acid molecule(s). Modern techniques of enzyme surgery permit the excision of a particular nucleotide sequence, e.g., within a nonessential gene, or ideally a gene conferring virulence [*Lai* et al., 1980; *Chanock*, 1981; *Roizman* et al., 1982]. So far, 'virulence genes' have proved to be elusive [*Palese and Roizman*, 1980; *Richman and Murphy*, 1979], although there are indications that the TK gene may be required for pathogenicity [*Field and Wildy*, 1978] and for establishment of latency [*Tenser* et al., 1979] in herpes simplex. Painstaking examination of the biological properties of deletion mutants and of recombinants obtained by transfection of cloned recombinant cDNAs [*Nomoto* et al., 1982] might offer a technological approach to defining the functions, including those relating to virulence, not only of individual viral genes but of sequences within those genes.

C. Recombinants Incorporating Cloned Genes from Other Viruses

Moss and his colleagues have recently opened up a novel approach to vaccination which may prove to be of widespread applicability [see *Smith* et al., 1983; *Panicali* et al., 1983]. The concept is to insert the gene for any given viral protein into the genome of an avirulent virus that can then be administered as a live vaccine. Cells in which the virus multiplies will produce the foreign viral protein, against which an immune response will then be mounted.

The prototype developed by *Smith* et al. [1983] is a 'live' vaccine in which the gene for hepatitis B surface antigen (HBsAg) is inserted into the genome of vaccinia virus. In brief, the recombinant was constructed as follows. The gene for HBsAg was inserted, within a nonessential vaccinia viral gene (e.g., that for thymidine kinase, TK), into a bacterial plasmid. A vaccinia early promoter was placed in the appropriate position adjacent to the 'foreign' (HBsAg) gene. Mammalian cells were then infected with wild-type vaccinia virus, and shortly thereafter transfected with the chimeric plasmid. Recombination occurred between the vaccinia DNA and the plasmid DNA. Appropriate selection procedures enabled recombinant vaccinia virions containing the HBsAg gene to be recovered. Following inoculation of such recombinants into cultured cells or rabbits, the virus multiplied and substantial quantities of HBsAg were secreted from infected cells. The animals produced an excellent antibody response to HBsAg. More recently, this vaccine has been shown to protect chimpanzees against challenge with hepatitis B, while analogous vaccinia-influenza (HA) and vaccinia-herpes simplex (gD) recombinants protected animals against influenza and herpes simplex, respectively [see *Smith* et al., and *Paoletti and Panicali* – in *Lerner and Chanock,* 1984].

This dramatic demonstration of the power of recombinant DNA technology is a real *tour de force.* In theory at least, it should now be possible to insert the gene for any, or indeed several, foreign proteins into the DNA of an avirulent live virus, such as vaccinia. Thereby one could hope to vaccinate simultaneously against a whole range of infectious diseases, including not only those of viral etiology but also perhaps malaria and other scourges of mankind. The potential benefits, particularly to the Third World, are self-evident.

Vaccinia virus may not necessarily turn out to be the ideal vector as many people are already immune and, furthermore, the vaccine is not absolutely safe [*Fenner,* 1982]. Perhaps a non-oncogenic adenovirus would be a suitable alternative. Or it may prove possible to manipulate the vaccinia viral genome to reduce its undesirable side-effects, particularly encephalitis. It may become necessary to develop several alternative vectors because, once a particular virus has been used, it cannot be reused as a live vaccine to immunize against another agent in the future. Alternatively, careful thought may need to be given to the construction of a single one-off, all-purpose vaccine incorporating genes for the key immunogenic proteins of most or all of the important human infectious diseases before substantial numbers of people are vaccinated with that vector in the first place.

D. 'Cloning'

The impact of recombinant DNA technology on vaccine design has been as striking as elsewhere. Already the complete genomes or selected genes of several mammalian viruses have been 'cloned' in bacteria, yeasts or mammalian cells using a range of plasmids, cosmids, phages and mammalian viral DNAs as vectors. Table VIII, which is certain to be incomplete by the time this monograph is published, lists those viral proteins that had, at the time of writing, been produced by recDNA technology, and

Table VIII. Some viral genes cloned by recombinant DNA technology

Virus	Gene	Vector	Host cell	Expression	Secretion	Reference
Hepatitis B	HBsAg	plasmid	*E. coli*	+	–	*Edman* et al. [1981]
	HBsAg	plasmid	*E. coli*	+	–	*Mackay* et al. [1981]
	HBsAg	phage λ	*E. coli*	+	–	*Charnay* et al. [1980]
	HBsAg	plasmid	*S. cerevisiae*	+	–	*Valenzuela* et al. [1982]
	HBsAg	plasmid	mouse Ltk^-	+	+	*Pourcel* et al. [1982]
	HBsAg	plasmid[a]	CV-1	+	+	*Smith* et al. [1983]
Herpes simplex 1	gD	plasmid	E. coli	+	–	*Weis* et al. [1983]
Influenza	HA	plasmid	E. coli	+	–	*Emtage* et al. [1980]
	HA	plasmid	E. coli	+	–	*Davis* et al. [1983]
	HA	SV40	MK	+	+	*Gething and Sambrook* [1981]
	HA	SV40	MK	+	+	*Sveda* et al. [1982]
Foot-and-mouth disease	VP1	plasmid	*E. coli*	+	–	*Küpper* et al. [1981]
	VP3	plasmid	*E. coli*	+	–	*Kleid* et al. [1981]
Poliomyelitis	complete genome	plasmid	CV-1, HeLa	+	+	*Racaniello and Baltimore* [1981]
Rabies	G	plasmid	E. coli	+	–	*Yelverton* et al. [1983]

[a] Chimeric plasmid incorporating foreign gene flanked by nonessential vaccina gene (e.g., TK) used to transfect mammalian cells co-infected with vaccinia virus; recombinant vaccinia virions containing gene for HBsAg selected for use as 'live' vaccine.

expressed in a form sufficiently immunogenic to be seriously considered as potential vaccines.

This is not the place to describe recombinant DNA technology, which has already mushroomed into a highly complex new specialty. The diversity of approaches to cloning in various prokaryotic and eukaryotic hosts using any of several types of vector occupy whole volumes [e.g., *Maniatis* et al., 1982]. Typical strategies are mentioned briefly under the heading of individual viral vaccines and are set out fully in the papers cited in table VIII as well as in a recent Cold Spring Harbor Symposium [*Lerner and Chanock,* 1984].

E. Synthetic Peptides

Three recent developments have opened up a radically new approach to vaccine design. Rapid methods for sequencing nucleic acids have led to the determination of the complete structure of the genome of a number of viruses [e.g., *Kitamura* et al., 1981], hence the amino acid sequence of the corresponding viral proteins can be simply read off (or determined directly) [*Laver and Air,* 1980]. Secondly, the tertiary structure of viral proteins can now be solved using X-ray crystallography [*Wilson* et al., 1981] and the antigenic sites identified by locating the position of amino acid substitutions in naturally occurring strains that have arisen by antigenic drift or in laboratory variants selected by monoclonal antibodies [*Wiley* et al., 1981; *Webster* et al., 1982]. Thirdly, the technology for synthesis of peptides in vitro has been refined and automated to the point where quite large quantities of such peptides can be synthesized chemically [*Sela and Arnon,* 1980; *Lerner,* 1982]. Hence one can now synthesize peptides corresponding to the critical antigenic determinants to which neutralizing antibodies bind.

It must be said that, in general, the neutralizing titer of antibodies induced by synthetic viral peptides is lower by orders of magnitude than that induced by inactivated vaccine, or even by the purified intact protein. This is not unexpected, as short peptides lack the original tertiary configuration of the antigenic determinant they represent [*Jackson* et al., 1981]; partial restoration of conformation by insertion of appropriately placed cross-linking bonds may partially restore immunogenicity [*Ionescu-Matiu* et al., 1983]. Furthermore, some 'conformational' determinants are 'non-sequential', i.e., are composed of amino acids that find themselves close together in the intact molecule but widely separated in the primary sequence [*Crumpton,* 1974]. Nevertheless, there are already some striking examples of synthetic viral peptides that have been shown to elicit neutralizing antibodies (e.g., hepatitis B [*Lerner* et al., 1981; *Ionescu-Matiu* et al., 1983]) and even to protect animals against challenge with a lethal dose of virus (foot-and-mouth-disease [*Bittle* et al., 1982]). Moreover, peptides incapable of inducing protective levels of antibody may nevertheless successfully prime an animal to respond anamnestically when subsequently boosted with a sub-immunizing dose of virus [*Emini* et al., 1983].

Most unexpected has been the observation that relatively invariate ('conserved'), even buried, amino acid sequences, that are evidently non-immunogenic under natural circumstances when presented as virus, may

Table IX. Synthetic peptides as potential vaccines

Virus	Reference
Hepatitis B	*Lerner* et al. [1981] *Dreesman* et al. [1982] *Hollinger* et al. [1982] *Prince* et al. [1982] *Gerin* et al. [1983] *Ionescu-Matiu* et al. [1983]
Influenza	*Jackson* et al. [1981, 1982] *Green* et al. [1982] *Müller* et al. [1982] *Lamb* et al. [1982] *Hackett* et al. [1983]
Foot-and-mouth disease	*Bittle* et al. [1982]
Poliomyelitis	*Emini* et al. [1983]
Herpes simplex	*Dietzschold* et al. [1984]

nevertheless, when presented as the isolated peptide, elicit antibodies that bind to virus and may even protect [*Lerner,* 1982]. Such conserved regions may be especially immunogenic for T lymphocytes and may have the unique advantage of eliciting cross-protection against heterologous serotypes of virus [*Anders* et al., 1981; *Lamb* et al., 1982; *Hackett* et al., 1983]. Table IX lists the key papers on synthetic viral peptides published at the time of writing.

F. Liposomes and Adjuvants

If isolated viral polypeptides – whether extracted from virions, mass-produced by recDNA technology, or synthesized chemically – are to be employed as vaccines, it is clear that their immunogenicity will need to be substantially augmented. Immunopotentiation can be accomplished with the help of adjuvants, carriers or liposomes.

Adjuvants such as aluminum phosphate and aluminum hydroxide gel to which the immunogen is adsorbed have been used safely in humans for many years, but the resulting immune response is not prolonged, hence booster injections are necessary. Concerns about potential carcinogenicity of nonmetabolizable adjuvants have held up progress in this area for the last couple of decades [*World Health Organization,* 1976]. More recently, attention has turned to simple, chemically defined, preferably synthetic substances of known mode of action. One of the most interesting is the active component of the Mycobacterium of Freund's complete adjuvant, namely the muramyl dipeptide (MDP), N-acetyl-muramyl-*L*-alanyl-*D*-isoglutamine [*Chedid* et al., 1976], and a non-pyrogenic MDP derivative [*Chedid* et al., 1982]. MDP and derivatives can be coupled to synthetic antigen [*Sela and Arnon,* 1980] or incorporated into liposomes [*Chedid,* 1979].

Recent extension of our understanding of lymphokines [*Feldmann and Schreier,* 1982; *Möller,* 1982b] raises the possibility that such molecules could potentially be used as adjuvants with specificity for particular subsets of lymphocytes [*Edelman* et al., 1980]. For instance, whereas an adjuvant that preferentially turned on suppressor T cells, T_d cells, IgE or the complement system may be disadvantageous or even disastrous, one that activated and/or mitogenized helper T cells and/or B cells might be extremely useful. Moreover, simple synthetic chemicals with these qualities might conceivably be conjugated to the immunogen in such a way that only the relevant clones of lymphocytes are activated.

Viral peptides can also be coupled to a carrier in order to elicit a more powerful helper T-cell response. For instance, the immunogenicity of foot-and-mouth disease virus peptides is enhanced by conjugation to keyhole limpet hemocyanin [*Bittle* et al., 1982]. If protein carriers were to be used in man it would be essential to exclude the possibility that on repeated administration they might precipitate hypersensitivity reactions.

Liposomes are micelles consisting of artificial lipid membranes into which proteins can be incorporated [*Gregoriadis,* 1976]. When purified viral envelope proteins are used, the resulting 'virosomes' (or 'immunosomes') somewhat resemble the original enveloped virion [*Simons* et al., 1978]. This ingenious trick enables one not only to reconstitute virus-like structures lacking all nucleic acid and other extraneous material, but also to select non-pyrogenic lipids and to incorporate substances with adjuvant activity, such as saponin or lipid A [*Naylor* et al., 1982], thus regaining much of the immunogenicity lost when the viral protein was removed from its original milieu [*Simons* et al., 1980].

XI. Human Viral Vaccines

The characteristics of the major human viral vaccines (tables X, XI) have been comprehensively reviewed [*Melnick,* 1977; *Horstmann,* 1979; *Hilleman,* 1980; *Meyer* et al., 1980; *Chanock,* 1981; *Sabin,* 1981a]. Accordingly, the ensuing summary will be confined to more recent developments. Readers seeking a fuller treatment are referred elsewhere [*Mims and White,* 1984].

A. Hepatitis

1. Hepatitis B

It is one of the great ironies that the most successful new vaccine to emerge in the past 5 years is against a virus we cannot yet grow in cultured cells. Such prodigious numbers of HBsAg particles circulate in the serum of hepatitis B carriers that they can be extracted directly from volunteers and, after purification and precautionary inactivation to destroy any possible contaminating live virus, used as a vaccine [*Maupas* et al., 1976; *Purcell and Gerin,* 1978; *Skelly* et al., 1981; reviews: *Vyas* et al., 1978; *Maupas and Guesry,* 1981; *Szmuness* et al., 1982]. The protocol for the preparation of the first vaccine licensed for general human use, in 1981 [*Hilleman* et al., 1982] is set out in table XII. In a well-controlled trial in male homosexuals by *Szmuness* et al. [1980], this vaccine, administered intramuscularly as three doses at 0, 1 and 6 months, was demonstrated to produce no untoward side effects (other than an occasional sore arm) and no hepatitis, but to induce antibodies and to reduce the incidence of subsequent disease (for a year or two at least) by over 95% in this high-risk population. A dose of 20 μg HBsAg is now standard [*Szmuness* et al., 1981a], but 40 μg is preferable for immunologically compromised individuals, and 10 μg suffices for young children. There is some difference of opinion about the cost-effectiveness and desirability of pretesting for antibody status before vaccinating. Except in certain high-risk populations,

Table X. Viral vaccines commonly used in man[a]

Disease	Vaccine strain	Cell substrate[b]	Attenuation	Inactivation[c]	Route[d]
Rabies	Pasteur	HEF	–	BPL or TBP	i.m. or i.d.
Yellow fever	17D	chick embryo	+	–	s.c.
Poliomyelitis	Sabin 1, 2, 3 (OPV)	HEF	+	–	oral
Measles	Schwarz	CEF	+	–	s.c.
Rubella	RA27/3 or Cendehill	HEF RK	+	–	s.c.
Mumps	Jeryl Lynn	CEF	+	–	s.c.
Influenza	A/H3N2, B (A/H1N1)	chick embryo	–	BPL or formalin or HANA subunits	i.m.
Hepatitis B	–[e]	–	–	HBsAg[e]	i.m.

[a] A wide variety of different viral strains and cell substrates are used in different countries; the selection listed is not comprehensive.
[b] CEF = Chick embryo fibroblast cultures; HEF = diploid strain of human embryonic fibroblasts; RK = rabbit kidney cultures.
[c] BPL = β-Propiolactone; TBP = tri-(n)-butylphosphate.
[d] i.m. = Intramuscular; i.d. = intradermal; s.c. = subcutaneous.
[e] Hepatitis B surface antigen purified from serum of human donors, then formalin-treated.

the incidence of anti-HBs is low in western countries. Carriers of HBsAg do not respond to the vaccine but are done no harm by it [*Dienstag* et al., 1982].

Of course the vaccine is expensive and will always be in short supply. Until it is supplanted by the next generation of hepatitis B vaccines, careful thought needs to be given to the priorities of its distribution in any given community or institution. High-risk target populations identified by the *Centers for Disease Control* [1982c] are set out in table XIII.

In an emergency, immediate protection can be conferred by giving immune human globulin at the same time as the first dose of vaccine [*Szmuness* et al., 1981b]. Such combined active-passive immunization could be advisable in the case of accidental exposure to contaminated blood, and in acutely infected or carrier pregnant women and their newborn babies.

In the longer term it will be necessary to replace this vaccine with something much more widely available if we are to contemplate routine

Table XI. Schedules for immunization against human viral diseases[a]

Vaccine	Primary course	Subsequent doses
Live vaccines		
Poliomyelitis	2–6 months of age, then 1 or 2 further doses at 2- to 3-month intervals[b]	school entry
Measles	12 months[c] (single dose)	–
Rubella	12 months[d] (single dose)	high school entry[d] (girls only)
Mumps	12 months (single dose)	–
Yellow fever	before travel to endemic area	10 years
Inactivated vaccines		
Influenza	autumn[e]	annual booster
Rabies	after bite, then at 3, 7, 14 and 28 days	–
Hepatitis B	when at risk[f], then 1 and 6 months later	?

[a] Schedules vary from country to country. This table is to be taken only as a guide.
[b] Two or three doses spaced 2 months apart during 1st year of life, commencing between 2 and 6 months of age. A further dose at 15–18 months is not essential but should be given if there is any doubt about whether the first three doses were received.
[c] Given on or shortly after 1st birthday in most developed countries, but as early as 6–9 months in some tropical developing countries where measles death rate is high in the second 6 months of life.
[d] Current US policy is to immunize males and females shortly after 1st birthday. Current UK policy is to immunize females only, on entry into high school. Recommended here is a combination of both.
[e] Vulnerable groups only, e.g., old respiratory invalids.
[f] Vulnerable groups only, e.g., family contacts and babies of carriers, patients and staff of hemodialysis units, blood banks, laboratories, hospitals, institutions for mentally retarded, etc., immunosuppressed, drug addicts, male homosexuals.

immunization of all infants in those areas of Asia, Africa and Oceania where the infection is so prevalent. A conventional live attenuated or inactivated vaccine is likely to be highly satisfactory and should follow within a few years of the growth of the virus in cell culture. The cross-protection between subtypes reported with the existing HBsAg vaccines and with cross-challenge experiments in chimpanzees seems to be of sufficient magnitude to obviate the necessity to include more than one virus in such a vaccine.

Table XII. Steps in the preparation of a human hepatitis B vaccine[a]

1. Collect plasma by regular plasmapheresis of known high titer HBsAg human carriers negative for infectious virions (Dane particles), DNA polymerase and HBeAg
2. Defibrinate with calcium
3. Concentrate HBsAg by precipitation with ammonium sulfate
4. Band by isopycnic (equilibrum) ultracentrifugation in sodium bromide
5. Reband by rate zonal centrifugation in sucrose gradient
6. Treat with pepsin, pH 2, to digest adsorbed plasma and liver proteins
7. Denature with 8 *M* urea, then renature (also to remove extraneous proteins)
8. Purify by gel (molecular sieve) filtration
9. Treat with formalin, 1:4,000, 3 days to inactivate any residual infectious virus
10. Adsorb onto aluminum hydroxide as adjuvant (0.5 mg alum per 20 μg HBsAg) and add thimerosal 1:20,000 as preservative
11. Ampoule in 1-ml doses (20 μg HBsAg) and store at 4 °C

[a] Reproduced in modified form from *Hilleman* et al. [1982].

Table XIII. Candidates for hepatitis B vaccine

Family contacts of known chronic HBsAg carriers
Babies born of HBeAg-positive mothers
Patients with diseases requiring frequent transfusions
Patients and staff of hemodialysis units
Medical and ancillary personnel in other high-risk situations, e.g., blood banks, serology laboratories, dental surgery, surgery, pathology
Inmates and staff of homes for the mentally retarded and other custodial institutions
Immunosuppressed or cancer patients
Drug addicts
Male homosexuals and prostitutes

Meanwhile, some are interested in the possibility that HBsAg could be obtained safely in commercial quantities from a human hepatoma cell line [*Alexander* et al., 1978]. Furthermore, hepatitis B DNA has been cloned in *E. coli* [*Burrell* et al., 1979] and sufficient expression of HBsAg obtained [*Charnay* et al., 1980; *Edman* et al., 1981; *Mackay* et al., 1981] to engender some optimism that this may be the way to go. Yields of immunogenic HBsAg are substantially greater from transfected mammalian cells [*Pourcel* et al., 1982; see also *Lerner and Chanock,* 1984], or from yeast, in which morphologically typical HBsAg particles are made [*Valenzuela* et al.,

1982; *Miyanohara* et al., 1983]. Moreover, following the demonstration that individual polypeptides derived from HBsAg are immunogenic [*Sanchez* et al., 1980; *Hollinger* et al., 1982], *Lerner* et al. [1981], *Dreesman* et al. [1982], *Prince* et al. [1982], and *Gerin* et al. [1983] have synthesized shorter peptides which are themselves immunogenic, though much less so than the HBsAg particles produced by yeast or mammalian cells. Incorporation of synthetic polypeptides into micelles [*Skelly* et al., 1981], or cross-linking to restore conformation [*Ionescu-Matiu* et al., 1983], might restore immunogenicity to something like its original level. The exciting new approach recently introduced by *Moss* and colleagues in which recombinant vaccinia virus incorporating the gene for HBsAg is used as a 'live' vaccine to immunize against hepatitis B [*Smith* et al., 1983] was discussed earlier.

2. Hepatitis A

Now that hepatitis A virus has finally been cultured unequivocally in vitro [*Daemer* et al., 1981; *Provost* et al., 1981], the way is open to develop a vaccine against this common and widespread disease also. The feasibility of a hepatitis A vaccine has already been established in marmosets [*Provost and Hilleman,* 1978]. Virus isolated in fetal rhesus monkey kidney cell cultures has been adapted to human embryonic lung fibroblasts, but the yields are low [*Hilleman* et al., 1981a]. Nevertheless, attenuated virus derived by serial passage in these cells has been shown to protect marmosets against challenge with virulent hepatitis A [*Provost* et al., 1982]. Furthermore, serially passaged virus of the HM/175 strain derived by *Daemer* et al. [1981] appears to be avirulent yet immunogenic in chimpanzees [*Purcell* et al., personal commun.], hence could constitute satisfactory seed for preparation of an experimental vaccine to be tested in man.

B. Herpesviruses

In view of the ubiquity of the four herpesviruses of man and the amount of human suffering they cause, it may seem paradoxical that the development of vaccines against them has lagged so far behind. There are basically two reasons for this [*Parks and Rapp,* 1975]. Firstly, all except herpes simplex virus tend to remain cell-associated in culture, hence are difficult to purify in the quantities required for the production of an inactivated vaccine. On the other hand, many virologists are naturally wary about the prospect of live herpesvirus vaccines, lest they establish life-long persistent infections with unknown consequences, conceivably including cancer. Yet there are theoretical reasons for advocating live herpes vaccines because of the dominant role of cell-mediated immunity in the response to herpes infections, and such a vaccine has proven to be notably successful in the prevention of Marek's disease in chickens [*Purchase,* 1976].

1. Varicella-Zoster

Takahashi and his colleagues in Japan [reviews: *Takahashi* et al., 1981; *Gershon,* 1980] produced a live attenuated varicella vaccine, the OKA strain, by serial passage in human and guinea pig cells. The vaccine was tested not only in normal individuals but also in immunocompromised children suffering from such debilitating conditions as leukemia and nephrotic syndrome, who are seen as the principal target group for vaccination if it can be shown to be safe in them. Seroconversion occurred in 98% of normal recipients, and side effects (mild fever and papular rash) were observed only very occasionally. In the immunocompromised group, however, a significant minority developed mild varicella, particularly if their immunosuppressive drugs were not suspended for vaccination. In both populations, immunization conferred substantial protection against natural varicella [*Asano and Takahashi,* 1977]. More recently, *Neff* et al. [1981] have reported similarly encouraging results with their KMcC strain of varicella virus attenuated by 50 passages in WI-38 cells.

2. Cytomegalovirus

Cytomegalovirus (CMV), though not a major cause of morbidity in healthy people, is highly dangerous in two particular circumstances: it is the commonest infectious cause of mental retardation (cytomegalic inclusion disease) and the commonest infectious cause of death in bone marrow transplant recipients and other profoundly immunosuppressed patients [*Lang,* 1980; *Osborn,* 1981]. *Elek and Stern* [1974] were the first to develop an experimental vaccine against human CMV. Their strain Ad-169, attenuated by 54 passages in human embryonic fibroblasts, produced antibody following subcutaneous injection; the only side effect seemed to be a rather regular tendency to a delayed local reaction at the injection site. These findings were subsequently confirmed and extended by *Neff* et al. [1979]. Meanwhile, *Plotkin* and colleagues produced their Towne-125 strain by 125 passages in WI-38 and demonstrated both humoral and cellular immune responses in normal recipients; responses in patients being prepared for renal transplants were often much reduced or delayed [*Starr* et al., 1981]. A majority of the latter group were found to be excreting CMV in their urine following subsequent renal transplantation, thus raising doubts about the vaccine's efficacy or safety or both [*Osborn,* 1981].

3. EB Virus

EB virus is the etiological agent not only of the ubiquitous disease infectious mononucleosis but also, in all probability, of two highly malignant tumors, Burkitt lymphoma and nasopharyngeal carcinoma [*Epstein and Achong,* 1979]. *Epstein* has advocated the development of a vaccine, even though the virus cannot yet be grown in conventional cell culture. The 340,000-dalton glycoprotein component of the EB virus-induced membrane antigen complex has been extracted from a marmoset lymphoblastoid cell line, then incorporated into liposomes and demonstrated to induce EBV-neutralizing antibodies in mice [*North* et al., 1982] and marmosets [*Epstein* et al., 1983].

4. Herpes Simplex

Oddly enough, the only human herpesvirus that grows rapidly to high titer in culture and the one responsible for by far the greatest morbidity, namely herpes simplex, has not attracted as much attention until recently. Interest has been reawakened by the explosive increase in herpes genitalis. An experimental 'subunit' HSV type 2 vaccine, consisting of formaldehyde-treated viral glycoprotein adsorbed to alum adjuvant [*Hilleman* et al., 1981b] is currently under trial. Meanwhile, *Naylor* et al. [1982] have shown that antibody responses of mice to HSV-1 glycoproteins are greatly enhanced by incorporation of the immunogen into liposomes containing lipid A. Recently, *Watson* et al. [1982] have cloned the gene for the HSV-1 glycoprotein gD in *E. coli,* and the same group [*Weis* et al., 1983] have obtained greatly enhanced expression by constructing a hybrid gene encoding a chimeric protein containing HSV-1 gD, bacteriophage λ Cro and *E. coli* β-galactosidase; the chimeric protein elicits antibodies which neutralize the infectivity of both HSV-1 and HSV-2. The incorporation of the gD gene into vaccinia virus has been mentioned earlier. *Dietzschold* et al. [1984] have recently presented evidence for protection of mice by a synthetic HSV peptide. *Roizman* et al. [1982] have constructed live attenuated HSV-1/HSV-2 recombinants and live deletion mutants lacking a nonessential early gene; neither safety nor protection against challenge by a natural route of infection has yet been demonstrated.

C. Rabies

The human diploid cell vaccine (HDCV) developed at the Wistar Institute [*Wiktor* et al., 1978; *Plotkin,* 1980] has now supplanted all previous rabies vaccines. Grown in WI-38 or MRC-5 cell strains, the virus is concentrated, then inactivated with β-propiolactone, or with tri-(n) butylphosphate which 'splits' the virus into 'subunits'. The typical post-exposure immunization course, consisting of five intramuscular injections of HDCV spread over 1 month, together with a single dose of rabies hyperimmune globulin on day 0 [*Centers for Disease Control,* 1980b], has proven to be spectacularly successful – none of some hundreds of people vaccinated following the bite of proven rabid animals in Iran, Germany and the USA up till 1980 developed rabies [*Plotkin,* 1980; *Anderson* et al., 1980]. There was no evidence of the anaphylactic reactions or neurological sequelae for which earlier rabies vaccines were notorious – merely local and mild systemic reactions in about 20% of recipients. Subsequent work suggests that intradermal injection may reduce these trivial side effects even further, as well as effecting considerable savings. Costs may also be reduced by the Merieux Institute technique of growing the vaccine virus in Vero cells on microcarriers in suspension culture.

More recently, *Wiktor and Koprowski* [1982] have detected previously unrecognized strain differences in rabies viruses isolated from different areas of the world and attribute recent vaccine failures to such variants; they see a possible need to broaden the antigenic repertoire of future rabies vaccines. *Coulon* et al. [1983] have been able to select avirulent rabies mutants by growing virus in the presence of particular monoclonal antibodies; this could be developed as a useful general approach to the attenuation of viruses for possible use as live vaccines. Meanwhile, a genetically engineered vaccine looks distinctly feasible following the cloning of the gene representing the membrane glycoprotein of rabies virus [*Yelverton* et al., 1983], although protection of experimental animals has yet to be demonstrated [*Wunner* et al., 1983].

D. Respiratory Viruses

1. Influenza

A particularly serious complication, the Guillain-Barré syndrome, was encountered in one of every 10^5 Americans vaccinated against 'swine flu', i.e., A/New Jersey/76 (H1N1), during a mass campaign in 1976–1977 [*Schonberger* et al., 1979], but no such association has been reported with any subsequent influenza vaccine [*Centers for Disease Control,* 1981]. A more significant problem in the long term is the low level of protection conferred by inactivated influenza vaccines: at best about 70% for 1–2 years following immunization with the latest strain of influenza, but often much lower in the most important target group, the elderly [reviews: *Perkins and Regamey,* 1977; *Tyrrell and Smith,* 1979; *Dowdle,* 1981; *Tyrrell* et al., 1981; *Potter,* 1982]. Furthermore, our best efforts can be sabotaged by 'original antigenic sin'. The problem is well illustrated by the finding of *Hoskins* et al. [1979] that immunization of schoolchildren with a vaccine against the current influenza strain provided no protection in those immunized annually for a number of years with the most up-to-date vaccine.

There are a number of recent developments which could lead to an improved vaccine. Firstly, liposomes [*Gregoriadis,* 1976] containing hemagglutinin (HA) and neuraminidase (NA) induce a good immune response experimentally [*Brand,* personal commun.]. Secondly, a cDNA copy of the (RNA) gene for HA has been cloned, first in *E. coli* [*Emtage* et al., 1980], then in monkey cells [*Gething and Sambrook,* 1981; *Sveda and Lai,* 1981] from which secretion was ensured by deletion of the cDNA coding for the hydrophobic C-terminus of HA [*Sveda* et al., 1982]. HA produced by cloning is less immunogenic than that produced by conventional means [*Davis* et al., 1983], but it could be cheaper. Thirdly, the HA gene has been incorporated by recombination into the genome of vaccinia virus; vaccinated animals develop neutralizing antibodies and resist intranasal challenge with influenza [*Paoletti and Panicali; Smith* et al., in *Lerner and Chanock,* 1984]. Fourthly, antigenic peptides have been synthesized de novo [*Jackson* et al., 1981, 1982; *Green* et al., 1982; *Müller* et al., 1982]. Strangely, the most immunogenic of these do not correspond with the known or presumptive antibody-binding sites on the HA molecule [*Wiley* et al., 1981; *Webster* et al., 1982; *Laver and Air,* 1980] but with relatively 'conserved' sequences that do not appear to be immunogenic in the intact virion [*Green* et al., 1982; *Müller* et al., 1982]. As mentioned earlier, some of these conserved regions of the molecule are more readily recognized by T cells and elicit a broadly reactive response [*Anders* et al., 1981; *Lamb* et al., 1982; *Hackett* et al., 1983].

There, are, however, good reasons for supposing that live vaccines may represent a superior alternative to all the options discussed so far

[*Chanock* et al., 1975; *Ada* et al., 1981; *Askonas* et al., 1982]. Live vaccines, empirically derived by serial passage in embryonated eggs and delivered intranasally, have been used for decades in the USSR, and during the 1970s on an experimental basis in Britain [*Beare,* 1975]. Systematic efforts to develop temperature-sensitive *(ts)* mutants as live influenza vaccines [reviews: *Chanock and Murphy,* 1980; *Murphy and Chanock,* 1981] were plagued by reversion towards virulence in man; in one revertant closely analyzed, at least three mutations had emerged, at least one of which did not display the characteristics of a simple reversion but was a suppressor mutation in the P2 gene that corrected the *ts* phenotype of the P3 gene product [*Murphy* et al., 1980].

Mention has been made of *Maassab's* cold-adapted *(ca)* mutants of influenza A/Ann Arbor/60 (H2N2) which are avirulent for ferrets, grow as well at 25 as at 33 °C and are also *ts,* with a ceiling temperature of 37 °C. Reassortants containing 6 *ca* genes from the master (donor) strain and only the HA and NA genes from the recipient wild-type strain, are *ca, ts* and highly attenuated for man when administered intranasally. Clinical trials currently underway indicate that these *ca* recombinants revert only rarely and partially, hence seem to be promising candidates for more general introduction as live attenuated intranasal vaccines [*Maassab* et al., 1981; *Murphy and Chanock,* 1981; *Kendal* et al., 1982; *Wright* et al., 1982].

Recently, *Murphy* et al. [1982], reasoning that a reassortant containing six genes derived from an avian influenza strain might be avirulent but immunogenic in man, have demonstrated that such a reassortant delivered transtracheally to monkeys is in fact protective; preliminary human trials [*Murphy* et al., personal commun.] indicate that the reassortant multiplies satisfactorily in the upper respiratory tract without symptoms.

2. Respiratory Syncytial Virus (RSV)

Following the discovery that an experimental inactivated RSV vaccine actually predisposed children to suffer more severe disease than unimmunized controls following a subsequent epidemic [*Chanock* et al., 1968; *Merz* et al., 1980], *Chanock* and colleagues redirected their efforts towards the development of an intranasal *ts* live vaccine. But even those *ts* mutants that contained multiple changes induced by the mutagen nitrosoguanidine and were shown to be attenuated for hamsters and chimpanzees proved not to be completely stable in vivo [*Chanock and Murphy,* 1980]. So this approach was also abandoned. Nevertheless, valuable data have been obtained which may influence the design of future live respi-

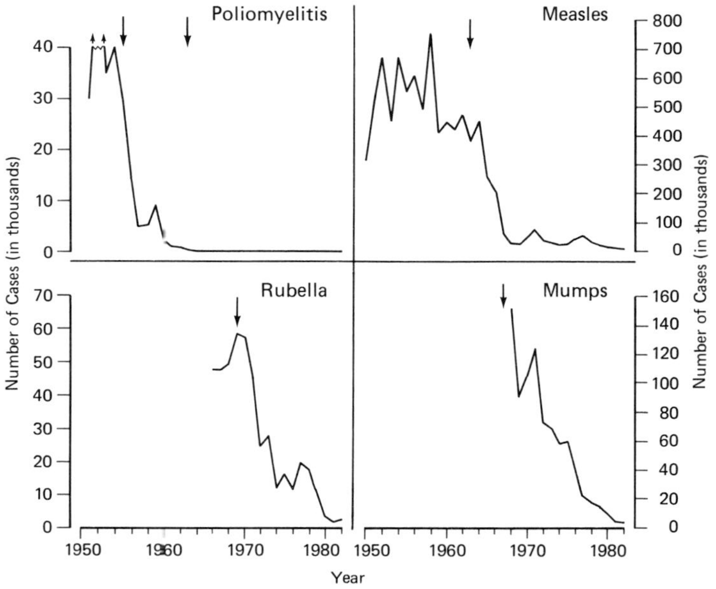

Fig. 5. Annual incidence of various viral diseases in the USA: date of introduction of vaccine indicated by arrow. (Compiled from data kindly supplied by the Centers for Disease Control.)

ratory viral vaccines [*Tyeryar* et al., 1978]. For instance, *Prince, Chanock* et al. [personal commun.] have shown that live RSV vaccine gives durable protection of hamsters and cotton rats against pneumonitis but not against rhinitis, leading them to postulate a qualitative, not simply quantitative, distinction between 'pulmonary immunity' and 'nasal immunity'.

E. Old Vaccines – New Developments

1. Poliomyelitis

The dramatic decline in the incidence of paralytic poliomyelitis that followed the introduction, first of inactivated polio vaccine (IPV), then shortly thereafter of live attenuated oral vaccine (OPV) (fig. 5) represents one of the great achievements of medical science. All aspects of immunization against polio have been comprehensively reviewed [*Sabin,* 1980, 1981; *Salk and Salk,* 1977; *Melnick,* 1978, 1980; *Horstmann,* 1979]. Accordingly, we will confine our attention to relatively recent developments.

In stark contrast to the spectacular success of the polio vaccination programs of the wealthy countries in temperate climates, relatively little impact has been made on the disease throughout most of the Third World [*Sabin* 1981b]. The reasons for this are complex but go mainly to the lack of adequate health service infrastructure. Many children in rural areas never receive a full course of OPV, and even when they do there are doubts about whether the viability of the virus has been retained by adequate refrigeration during storage and transport in hot tropical climates. Maintenance of the 'cold chain' is therefore of vital importance [*Assaad,* 1979; *Sabin,* 1980], and molar $MgCl_2$ also helps to stabilize the vaccine [*Melnick,* 1978]. It has been suggested that much more extensive coverage can be obtained by annual mass immunization campaigns aimed at all children under the age of, say, 3 to 5 years, on 2 nominated days 2 months apart [*Borgono* et al., 1980; *Sabin,* 1980, 1981b]. There is a case for using only type 1 for the first dose (and also in the face of a known type 1 epidemic) as at least 85% of paralytic cases are attributable to this serotype [*Sabin,* 1980]. That polio can indeed be almost eradicated by comprehensive coverage with OPV in tropical countries has been amply demonstrated by the superb record of Brazil, Chile and Cuba, to name three particularly impressive examples [*Borgono* et al., 1980; *Sabin,* 1980]. Eradication of poliomyelitis from the Third World is a major objective of WHO's Expanded Programme of Immunization (EPI) [*Assaad,* 1979; *Sabin,* 1980, 1981b].

In the more advanced nations, where the disease has been effectively conquered, it remains imperative that very high levels of immunization are maintained in spite of the lack of perceived threat. Pockets of unimmunized people, e.g., immigrants concentrated in urban ghettos, are particularly vulnerable to imported viruses. Similarly, outbreaks occurred among the Arab population of Gaza and the West Bank of the Jordan during the 1970s [*Melnick,* 1980]. Another recent salutary experience was the outbreak of poliomyelitis in 1978 in Holland which was confined entirely to members of a particular religious minority who had refused immunization. The epidemic spread to Canada and then to the USA where it affected only unimmunized members of the Amish community, causing many cases of paralysis [*Melnick,* 1980].

Such has been the success of OPV in the USA that about half of the minuscule number of cases of paralytic poliomyelitis that still occur are 'vaccine-associated'. The precise incidence is difficult to ascertain as some cases may not in fact be polio [*Sabin,* 1981b], but the upper limit appears to be about 1 case per million vaccinees [*Nightingale,* 1977; *Nathanson and*

Martin, 1979; *Moore* et al., 1982; *WHO Consultative Group,* 1982]. Immunocompromised individuals are up to 10,000 times more vulnerable than normal [*Melnick,* 1980]. Most vaccine-associated cases are due to the type 3 component of the vaccine, or type 2, especially in unimmunized family contacts. No doubt the fact that vaccine strains, excreted in feces, can spread to nonimmune contacts [*Fox and Hall,* 1980] increases the probability of emergence of mutants displaying varying degrees of reversion towards virulence [*Kew* et al., 1981; *Nakano* et al., 1978].

The occurrence of these rare 'vaccine-associated' cases of paralysis is being used by some as an argument for returning to IPV [*Salk and Salk,* 1977; *D. Salk,* 1980; *Hennessen and van Wezel,* 1981]. But this is probably an overreaction. By any objective measure OPV is one of the safest vaccines ever developed. Nevertheless, certain refinements of the present OPV policy are called for and have recently been recommended for general implementation in the USA [*Nightingale,* 1977; *Centers for Disease Control,* 1982a]. Firstly, IPV should be preferred in anyone known to be immunocompromised. Secondly, because there are still significant numbers of parents who have never received polio vaccine, there are good arguments for immunizing such nonimmune family contacts prior to or simultaneously with their infants [*Melnick,* 1978, 1980], as well as for routine boosters for every child at 1 year, then on entering school, and again on entering high school [*Nightingale,* 1977]. Thirdly, it has been recommended that nonimmunized adults traveling to developing countries where polio is still endemic should receive IPV rather than OPV because of the slightly higher risk of OPV-associated polio in adults; however, the data on this latter point are marginal and the established dogma that nonimmune adults are more prone to paralysis by wild poliovirus than are young children has been cogently challenged [*Nathanson and Martin,* 1979].

IPV of greater potency is now being produced as a result of a number of technological improvements [*Hennessen and van Wezel,* 1981]. Since many species of monkeys are declared to be endangered and cannot lawfully be exported from their countries of origin, they are now bred in captivity and can be more effectively screened for adventitious herpes B and 'foamy' viruses. Furthermore, cynomolgus monkey kidney cells can now be subcultured for a few generations and grown on the surface of myriads of DEAE-Sephadex beads known as 'microcarriers' suspended in large fermentation tanks [*van Wezel* et al., 1978]. Unfortunately, human diploid cell strains, which have tended to replace primary cultures of monkey kidney as the substrate for production of OPV and most other human viral vaccines in recent years [*Plotkin,* 1980], do not grow sufficiently well to make them a commercial proposition for production of the very large amounts of virus required for IPV, but nonmalignant, aneuploid monkey kidney cell lines such as Vero, LLC-MK_2 or CV-1 [*Montagnon* et al., 1981; *Petricciani* et al., 1979] have recently been approved for this purpose. Following clarification, virus is purified from the supernatant by gel filtration and ion exchange chromatography, e.g., on DEAE-Sepharose 6B, or affinity chromatography on Sepharose 4B-immobilized antibodies, and/or zonal ultracentrifugation [*van Wezel,* 1981]. Two doses of the newer preparations of IPV appear to confer protection equivalent to the four previously required. This has encouraged the proposal that IPV replace OPV, particularly in the Third World, where unsatisfactory seroconversion rates are frequently reported even after the full course of 3 doses of OPV. It would be convenient to incorporate IPV in the 'triple vaccine' (against diphtheria, pertussis and tetanus) which is already used routinely in most countries [*D. Salk,* 1980; *Hennessen and van Wezel,* 1981; *Beale,* 1982].

2. Measles

Immunization of children at the age of 12–15 months with the 'further-attenuated' live measles vaccine is now routine in many western countries [reviews: *Krugman,* 1977; *Centers for Disease Control,* 1982b]. Indeed, in the USA, where immunization is a legal precondition for school entry in most states [*Robbins* et al., 1981], indigenous measles has essentially disappeared [*Hinman* et al., 1980] (see also fig. 5). Many of the cases that still occur follow importations from abroad. As expected, the age distribution has shifted upwards and eradication of the disease will require more comprehensive immunization of older children and young adults as well as infants, at least for a 'catch-up' period of a decade or so.

In the developing countries of the tropics, where measles ranks with gastroenteritis and pneumonia as the major causes of death in malnourished infants [*Morley,* 1980; *Walsh and Warren,* 1979], immunization is a top priority. Maintenance of the cold chain is important; the freeze-dried vaccine stores well at 4 °C but after reconstitution is particularly vulnerable to inactivation by heat and light [*McAleer* et al., 1980]. The optimum age of immunization is the subject of debate and may differ from country to country depending upon the extent of protein malnutrition and age/mortality statistics. *Black* [1982] points out that seroconversion occurs in over

95% of 15-month-old recipients, but in only 50–75% at 6 months, yet the mortality in some tropical countries is so high that immunization as early as 9 (or even 6) months may be desirable. *Sabin* et al. [1983] have recently reported immunization of children, including 4–6 month olds possessing substantial levels of maternal antibody, by a live attenuated measles vaccine delivered as an aerosol from a nebulizer via a face mask.

3. Rubella

The original live attenuated rubella strain, HPV-77, has now been withdrawn, leaving the market to the human diploid-cell-grown RA27/3 and the rabbit kidney-grown Cendehill-51 [reviews: *Krugman,* 1977; *Horstmann,* 1979; *Preblud* et al., 1980]. Both provide satisfactory immunity, which is probably reinforced by subclinical infection that may occur a few years later as antibody levels decline.

Arthralgia, seen mainly in adult females and usually confined to the small peripheral joints, is still a not uncommon side effect of both vaccines [*Preblud* et al., 1980]. Rarely, this may progress to frank arthritis, which may persist for years with recurrent exacerbations during which virus may be isolated from lymphocytes [*Chantler* et al., 1981]. Another rare complication is peripheral neuritis [*Preblud* et al., 1980]. There is still no evidence that the vaccine virus is teratogenic [*Preblud* et al., 1981]. Hence, accidental immunization during pregnancy is not considered to be an indication for termination [*Centers for Disease Control,* 1981]. Nevertheless, since the vaccine virus is known to cross the placenta and infect the fetus, prudence suggests that women not be deliberately immunized during the first trimester and that nonpregnant vaccinees should be advised to avoid conception for the next 2–3 months, and/or should be immunized immediately postpartum [*Preblud* et al., 1980].

From the outset in 1969, two opposing schools of thought have dictated the strategies of rubella vaccine programs in different parts of the world. In the UK and Australia, for example, the primary target population has been teenage females; the policy has been to immunize all girls on entry into high school (i.e., usually 12–13 years of age). By contrast, the USA have aimed to immunize all children, male and female, early in the 2nd year of life. An ancillary feature of both policies has been to immunize seronegative females of childbearing age.

Neither strategy can be deemed an unqualified success [*Knox,* 1980; *Preblud* et al., 1980]. As would be expected from the fact that rubella circulates mainly among children of preschool and primary school age, the

UK program has had no demonstrable effect on the overall incidence of rubella; more disturbingly, however, it has not yet apparently led to a major decline in the incidence of the congenital rubella syndrome (CRS), probably because the coverage of teenage girls has been inadequate and most women in the age group 25–45 years have been missed entirely [*Dudgeon*, 1979; *Preblud* et al., 1980]. The US program, on the other hand, has led to a substantial decline in the incidence of rubella in children, but not in adolescents or adults, and has had only a modest impact on the occurrence of CRS [*Krugman*, 1977; *Preblud* et al., 1980]. This too is not unexpected as the cohort at which the vaccine was targeted during the 1970s is only now moving into the childbearing years.

These worrying findings suggest the following course of action. Firstly, careful studies must be undertaken to determine the level and duration of immunity up to 40 years after RA27/3 and Cendehill vaccines, in the absence as well as in the presence of natural subclinical booster infections. Secondly, vaccine uptake rate must be increased to at least 80–90%, whichever vaccination schedule is employed. Thirdly, the ideal strategy might be to ensure >90% coverage of 1-year-olds, male and female, coupled with a policy, for the next several years at least, of vigorous pursuit and immunization of nonimmune 15- to 40-year-old women. The foregoing has now been adopted as the revised rubella vaccination policy for the USA [*Centers for Disease Control*, 1981].

4. Mumps

Live mumps vaccine is now widely used in the USA, in combination with live attenuated measles and rubella [*Stokes* et al., 1971] at 12–15 months of age, or alone, particularly to adolescent males [*Centers for Disease Control*, 1980a]. Protective levels of antibody in at least 95% of recipients are conferred by a single subcutaneous injection and persist for at least a decade [*Weibel* et al., 1979]. A marked decline in the incidence of mumps has occurred in the USA since the introduction of the vaccine [*Hayden* et al., 1978] (see also fig. 5).

5. Arboviruses

The live attenuated vaccine against yellow fever, developed empirically years ago when virology was still in its infancy, is still one of the safest and most effective of all the vaccines in use today [*World Health Organization*, 1971; *Monath* et al., 1983], although there is certainly a case for updating the manufacturing procedures, e.g. to insist on specific-pathogen-free and leukosis-free chickens and to move towards exclusively cell culture (CEF)-grown vaccine [*World Health Organization,* 1983].

There is an evident need for vaccines against at least a dozen other arboviruses responsible for such devastating diseases as encephalitis and hemorrhagic fever in various parts of the world. In general, however, the pharmaceutical companies do not feel in a position to undertake the costly development and testing required for the production of vaccines against agents that are not prevalent in the affluent western world.

Nevertheless, some satisfactory vaccines are in use. For example, a formalin-inactivated, mouse-brain-derived Japanese encephalitis vaccine is routinely administered to Japanese children and has dramatically reduced the incidence of that disease in Japan [*Hammon* et al., 1971]. A more potent formalin-killed vaccine derived from virus grown in cultured hamster kidney cells has proved to be at least as efficacious as its predecessor $\geqq$80%) in field trials, and no encephalitis or other serious side-effects have so far been reported in vaccinees [*World Health Organization,* 1983]. However, like the mouse brain vaccine, it induces only short-lived immunity, hence regular boosters will be necessary. There is a good case also for routine immunization of the principal domestic animal host, the pig.

Another formalin-inactivated vaccine, against tick-borne encephalitis, is produced in chick embryonic fibroblast cultures, and administered to vulnerable populations in Eastern Europe as a primary course of injections followed by annual boosters. Improved, more concentrated versions of this vaccine, recently developed in the USSR and Austria, are reported to give 85–100% seroconversion following a single subcutaneous inoculation, to prevent paralysis and to reduce the incidence of meningoencephalitis [*World Health Organization,* 1983].

For some years a live vaccine (TC-83) has been used successfully for the protection of laboratory workers as well as horses against Venezuelan equine encephalitis; more recently, a formalin-inactivated vaccine (C-84) prepared from the attenuated TC-83 strain has been shown to be protective and safe [*Edelman* et al., 1979]. Inactivated vaccines are also available against Russian spring-summer encephalitis and Rift Valley fever.

The desirability of a vaccine against the most widespread of all the arboviral diseases, dengue fever, must be considered in the light of the current debate about the pathogenesis of dengue hemorrhagic fever/shock syndrome. If indeed the syndrome is the result of enhanced viral replication in the presence of antibody to a heterologous serotype ('immune infection enhancement' [*Halstead,* 1981]), then widespread active immunization against dengue could turn out to be a disaster unless protective levels of antibodies against all four types could be guaranteed for life. Nevertheless, *Russell* et al. [in preparation] have recently tested an experimental dengue type 2 vaccine in man.

Safety considerations impose restraints on laboratory work with many of the dangerous arboviruses, and more particularly the arenaviruses, rhabdoviruses and filoviruses. The most appropriate application of recombinant DNA technology to vaccine development may well turn out to be in this area.

Acknowledgements

I am particularly indebted to *Dr. R.M. Chanock* for his hospitality during my four months' study leave in his laboratory during which this review was written in late 1982. I am also most grateful to Professor *C.A. Mims* and to Blackwell of Oxford for permission to incorporate in the Vaccines section of this review some figures, tables and other material abstracted from a more extensive survey I had written for Mims & White: 'Viral Pathogenesis and Immunology'. For helpful discussions and/or the provision of preprints, acknowledgement is due to Drs. *C. Baglioni, J. Beale, R.M. Chanock, A. L. Cunningham, E. de Clercq, M.A. Epstein, F. Fenner, N.B. Finter, G.J. Galasso, D.V. Goeddel, M.R. Hilleman, A.E. Hinman, A.Z. Kapikian, H. Koprowski, I.M. Kerr, P. Lengyel, R.A. Lerner, J.L. Melnick, T.C. Merigan, B.R. Murphy, G. Noble, J.S. Oxford, S. Pestka, R.H. Purcell, M. Revel, A.B. Sabin, J. Vilček,* and *C. Weissmann.* Finally, I would like to thank Drs. *R.M. Chanock, F. Fenner, A.R. Hinman, C.A. Mims* and *B.R. Murphy* for their comments on the manuscript.

References

Ada, G. L.; Leung, K. N.; Ertl, H.: An analysis of effector T cell generation and function in mice exposed to influenza A or Sendai viruses. Immunol. Rev. *58:* 5 (1981).

Aguet, M.: High affinity binding of ^{125}I-labeled mouse interferon to a specific cell surface receptor. Nature, Lond. *284:* 459 (1980).

Alexander, J.; Macnab, G.; Saunders, R.: Studies on in vitro production of hepatitis B surface antigen by a human hepatoma cell line. Perspect. Virol. *10:* 103 (1978).

Allen, G.; Fantes, K. H.: A family of structural genes for human lymphoblastoid (leukocyte-type) interferon. Nature, Lond. *287:* 408 (1980).

Anders, E. M.; Katz, J. M.; Brown, L. E.; Jackson, D. C.; White, D. O.: The specificity of T cells for influenza virus hemagglutinin; in Nayak, Genetic variation among influenza viruses. ICN-UCLA Symp., vol. 21, pp. 547–565 (Academic Press, New York 1981).

Anderson, L. J.; Sikes, R. K.; Langkop, C. W.; Mann, J. M.; Smith, J. S.; Winkler, W. G.; Deitch, M. W.: Postexposure trial of a human diploid cell strain rabies vaccine. J. infect. Dis. *142:* 133 (1980).

Asano, Y.; Takahashi, M.: Clinical and serologic testing of a live varicella vaccine and two-year follow-up for immunity of the vaccinated children. Pediatrics, Springfield *60:* 810 (1977).

Ashton, W. T.; Karkas, J. D.; Field, A. K.; Tolman, R. L.: Activation by thymidine kinase and potent antiherpetic activity of 2′-nor-2′-deoxyguanosine (2′NDG). Biochem. biophys. Res. Commun. *108:* 1716 (1982).

Askonas, B. A.; McMichael, A. J.; Webster, R. G.: The immune response to influenza viruses and the problem of protection against infection; in Beare, Basic and applied influenza research, chapt. 7 (CRC Press, Cleveland 1982).

Assaad, F.: Poliomyelitis vaccination benefits versus risk. Dev. biol. Standard., vol. 43, p. 141 (Karger, Basel 1979).

Bader, J. P.; Brown, N. R.; Chiang, P. K.; Cantoni, G. L.: 3-Deazaadenosine, an inhibitor of adenosylhomocysteine hydrolase, inhibits reproduction of Rous sarcoma virus and transformation of chick embryo cells. Virology *89:* 494 (1978).

Baglioni, C.: Interferon-induced enzymatic activities and their role in the antiviral state. Cell *17:* 255 (1979).

Baglioni, C.: The molecular mediators of interferon action; in Came, Carter, Interferons and their applications, Handbook of experimental Pharmacology, vol. 71 (Springer, Berlin 1983).

Baglioni, C.; Minks, M. A.; Maroney, P. A.: Interferon action may be mediated by activation of a nuclease by pppA2′p5′A2′p5′A. Nature, Lond. *273:* 684 (1978).

Balfour, H. F.; McMonigal, K. A.; Bean, B.: Acyclovir therapy of varicella-zoster infections in immunocompromised patients. J. antimicrob. Chemother. *12:* suppl. B, p. 169 (1983).

Balkwill, F. R.: Interferons as cell-regulatory molecules. Cancer Immunol. Immunother. *7:* 7 (1979).

Balkwill, F. R.; Griffin, D. B.; Band, H. A.; Beverley, P. C. L.: Immune human lymphocytes produce an acid-labile α-interferon. J. exp. Med. *157:* 1059 (1983).

Ball, L. A.: 2′,5′-Oligoadenylate synthetase; in Boyer, The enzymes, vol. 15, pp. 281–313 (Academic Press, New York 1982).

Baron, S.; Brunell, P. A.; Grossberg, S. E.: Mechanisms of action and pharmacology: the immune and interferon systems; in Galasso, Antiviral agents and viral diseases of man, pp. 151–208 (Raven Press, New York 1979).

Baron, S.; Dianzani, F.; Stanton, G. J.: The interferon system: review to 1982. Parts 1 and 2. Tex. Rep. Biol. Med. *41* (Univ. Texas, Medical Branch, Galveston 1982).

Barranger, J. A.; Rapoport, S. I.; Fredericks, W. R.; Pentchev, P. G.; Macdermot, K. D.; Steusing, J. K.; Brady, R. O.: Modification of the blood-brain barrier: increased concentration and fate of enzymes entering the brain. Proc. natn. Acad. Sci. USA *76:* 481 (1979).

Bauer, D. J.: The specific treatment of virus diseases (University Park Press, Baltimore 1977).

Bauer, D. J.: The chemotherapy of herpesvirus infections; in Waterson, Recent advances in clinical virology, vol. 2, pp. 111–127 (Churchill Livingstone, Edinburgh 1980a).

Bauer, D. J.: Laboratory studies on acyclovir; in Collier, Oxford, Developments in antiviral therapy, pp. 43–51 (Academic Press, London 1980b).

Bauer, D. J.; Selway, J. W. T.; Batchelor, J. F.; Tisdale, M.; Caldwell, I. C.; Young, D. A. B.: 4′,6-Dichloroflavan (BW683C), a new anti-rhinovirus compound. Nature, Lond. *292:* 369 (1981).

Beale, J.: Control of poliomyelitis: killed or living vaccine; in Mackenzie, Viral diseases of S. E. Asia and the Western Pacific, pp. 405–414 (Academic Press, Sydney 1982).

Beare, J. S.: Live viruses for immunization against influenza. Prog. med. Virol., vol. 20, p. 49 (Karger, Basel 1975).

Becker, Y.: Antiviral drugs. Monogr. Virol., vol. 11 (Karger, Basel 1976).

Becker, Y. (ed.): Antiviral drugs and interferon: the molecular basis of their activity (Nijhoff, The Hague 1982).

Becker, Y.; Hadar, J.: Antivirals 1980 – an update. Prog. med. Virol., vol. 26, p. 1 (Karger, Basel 1980).

Berg, K.: Purification and characterization of murine and human interferons. Acta pathol. microbiol. scand., C, Immunol., suppl. 279 (1982).

Billiau, A.: Interferon therapy: pharmacokinetic and pharmacological aspects. Archs Virol. *67:* 121 (1981).

Bittle, J. L.; Houghten, R. A.; Alexander, H.; Shinnick, T. M.; Sutcliffe, J. G.; Lerner, R. A.; Rowlands, D. J.; Brown, F.: Protection against foot-and-mouth disease with a chemically synthesized peptide predicted from the viral nucleotide sequence. Nature, Lond. *298:* 30 (1982).

Black, F. L.: Problems encountered in measles immunization in developing countries; in Mackenzie, Viral diseases of S. E. Asia and the Western Pacific, pp. 297–307 (Academic Press, Sydney 1982).

Boezi, J. A.: The antiherpesvirus action of phosphonoacetate. Pharmacol. Ther. *4:* 231 (1979).

Borgono, J. M.; Vicent, P.; Toro, J.: Efficacy of live poliovirus vaccine in Latin America; in André, Potency and efficacy of vaccines, pp. 73–82 (Smith Kline-RIT, USA 1980).

Brack, C.; Nagata, S.; Mantei, N.; Weissmann, C.: Molecular analysis of the human interferon-α gene family. Gene *15:* 379 (1981).

Branca, A. A.; Baglioni, C.: Evidence that types I and II interferons have different receptors. Nature, Lond. *294:* 768 (1981).

Breinig, M. C.; Morahan, P. S.: Interferon inducers: polyanions and others; in Stringfellow, Interferon and interferon inducers, pp. 239–261 (Dekker, New York 1980).

Brigden, D.; Fiddian, P.; Rosling, A. E.; Ravenscroft, T.: Acyclovir – a review of the preclinical and early clinical data of a new antiherpes drug. Antiviral Res. *1:* 203 (1981).

Brigden, D.; Fowle, A.; Rosling, A.: Acyclovir, a new antiherpetic drug: early experience in man with systemically administered drug; in Collier, Oxford, Developments in antiviral therapy, pp. 53–62 (Academic Press, London 1980).

Bryson, Y. J.: Current status and prospects for oral acyclovir treatment of first episode and recurrent genital herpes simplex virus. J. antimicrob. Chemother. *12:* suppl. B, p. 61 (1983).

Buchanan, R. A.; Hess, F.: Vidarabine (Vira-A®): pharmacology and clinical experience. Pharmacol. Ther. *8:* 143 (1980).

Burke, D. C.; Meager, A.: Genetic control of interferon formation. Ann. N.Y. Acad. Sci. *350:* 179 (1980).

Burns, W. H.; Saral, R.; Santos, G. W.; Laskin, O. L.; Lietman, P. S.; McLaren, C.; Barry, D. W.: Isolation and characterisation of resistant herpes simplex virus after acyclovir therapy. Lancet *i:* 421 (1982).

Burns, W. H.; Wingard, J. R.; Bender, W. J.; Saral, R.: Thymidine kinase not required for antiviral activity of acyclovir against mouse cytomegalovirus. J. Virol. *39:* 889 (1981).

Burrell, C. J.; MacKay, P.; Greenway, P. J.; Hofschneider, P. H.; Murray, K.: Expression in *Escherichia coli* of hepatitis B virus DNA sequences cloned in plasmid pBR322. Nature, Lond. *279:* 43 (1979).

Caliguiri, L. A.; Tamm, I.: Guanidine and 2-(α-hydroxybenzyl)-benzimidazole (HBB): selective inhibitors of picornavirus multiplication; in Carter, Selective inhibitors of viral functions, pp. 257–293 (CRC Press, Cleveland 1973).

Came, P. E.; Caliguiri, L. A.: Chemotherapy of viral infections; in Handbook of experimental Pharmacology, vol. 61 (Springer, Berlin 1982).

Came, P. E.; Carter, W. A. (eds.): Interferons and their applications; Handbook of experimental Pharmacology, vol. 71 (Springer, Berlin 1983).

Cantell, K.; Hirvonen, S.; Kauppinen, H.-L.; Myllylä, G.: Production of interferon in human leucocytes from normal donors with the use of Sendai virus. Meth. Enzym. *78:* 29 (1981).

Carrasco, L.: Membrane leakiness after viral infection and a new approach to the development of antiviral agents. Nature, Lond. *272:* 694 (1978).

Carrasco, L.: Modification of membrane permeability induced by animal viruses early in infection. Virology *113:* 623 (1981).

Cayley, P. J.; Silverman, R. H.; Wreschner, D. H.; Knight, M.; Gilbert, C. S.; Brown, R. E.; Kerr, I. M.: The 2-5A system in interferon-treated and control cells; in Mozes, Cellular responses to molecular modulators, pp. 347–360 (Academic Press, New York 1981).

Centers for Disease Control: Mumps vaccine. Morbidity Mortality Wkly Rep. *29:* 87–94 (1980a).

Centers for Disease Control: Rabies prevention. Morbidity Mortality Wkly Rep. *29:* 265–280 (1980b).

Centers for Disease Control: Rubella prevention. Morbidity Mortality Wkly Rep. *30:* 37–47 (1981).

Centers for Disease Control: Poliomyelitis prevention. Morbidity Mortality Wkly Rep. *31:* 22 (1982a).

Centers for Disease Control: Measles prevention. Morbidity Mortality Wkly Rep. *31:* 217–231 (1982b).

Centers for Disease Control: Inactivated hepatitis B virus vaccine. Morbidity Mortality Wkly Rep. *31:* 317–328 (1982c).

Chanock, R.M.: Strategy for development of respiratory and gastrointestinal tract viral vaccines in the 1980s. J. infect. Dis. *143:* 364 (1981).

Chanock, R.M.; Murphy, B.R.: Use of temperature-sensitive and cold-adapted mutant viruses in immunoprophylaxis of acute respiratory tract diseases. Rev. infect. Dis. *2:* 421 (1980).

Chanock, R.M.; Parrott, R.H.; Kapikian, A.Z.; Kim, H.W.; Brandt, C.D.: Possible role of immunological factors in pathogenesis of RS virus lower respiratory tract disease. Perspect. Virol. *6:* 125 (1968).

Chanock, R.M.; Richman, D.D.; Murphy, B.R.; Spring, S.B.; Schnitzer, T.J.; Richardson, L.S.: Current approaches to viral immunoprophylaxis; in Notkins, Viral immunology and immunopathology, pp. 291–316 (Academic Press, New York 1975).

Chantler, J.K.; Ford, D.K.; Tingle, A.J.: Rubella-associated arthritis: rescue of rubella virus from peripheral blood lymphocytes two years postvaccination. Infect. Immunity *32:* 1274 (1981).

Charnay, P.; Gervais, M.; Louise, A.; Galibert, F.; Tiollais, P.: Biosynthesis of hepatitis B virus surface antigen in *Escherichia coli.* Nature, Lond. *286:* 893 (1980).

Chedid, L. (ed.): Immunomodulation I and II. Springer Semin. Immunopathol. *2:* 1–232 (1979).

Chedid, L.; Audibert, F.; Lefrancier, P.; Choay, J.; Lederer, E.: Modulation of the immune response by a synthetic adjuvant and analogs. Proc. natn. Acad. Sci. USA *73:* 2472 (1976).

Chedid, L.A.; Parant, M.A.; Audibert, F.M.; Riveau, G.J.; Parant, F.J.; Lederer, E.; Choay, J.P.; Lefrancier, P.L.: Biological activity of a new synthetic muramyl peptide adjuvant devoid of pyrogenicity. Infect. Immunity *35:* 417 (1982).

Chou, S.; Gallagher, J.G.; Merigan, T.C.: Controlled trial of intravenous acyclovir in heart-transplant patients with mucocutaneous herpes simplex infections. Lancet *i:* 1392 (1981).

Clemens, M.J.; Williams, B.R.G.: Inhibition of cell-free protein synthesis by pppA2′p5′A2′p5′A: a novel oligonucleotide synthesized by interferon-treated L cell extracts. Cell *13:* 565 (1978).

Coen, D.M.; Schaffer, P.A.: Two distinct loci confer resistance to acycloguanosine in herpes simplex virus type 1. Proc. natn. Acad. Sci. USA *77:* 2265 (1980).

Colby, B.M.; Furman, P.A.; Shaw, J.E.; Elion, G.B.; Pagano, J.S.: Phosphorylation of acyclovir [9-(2-hydroxyethoxymethyl)guanine] in Epstein-Barr virus-infected lymphoblastoid cell lines. J. Virol. *38:* 606 (1981).

Collier, L. H.; Oxford, J. (eds.): Developments in antiviral therapy (Academic Press, London 1980).

Corey, L.; Benedetti, J.; Critchlow, C.; Mertz, G.; Douglas, J.; Fife, K.; Fahnlander, A.; Remington, M. L.; Winter, C.; Dragavon, J.: Treatment of primary first-episode genital herpes simplex virus infections with acyclovir: results of topical, intravenous and oral therapy. J. antimicrob. Chemother. *12:* suppl. B, p. 79 (1983).

Corey, L.; Nahmias, A. J.; Guinan, M. E.; Benedetti, J. K.; Critchlow, C. W.; Holmes, K. K.: A trial of topical acyclovir in genital herpes simplex virus infection. New Engl. J. Med. *306:* 1313 (1982).

Couch, R. B.; Jackson, G. G.: Antiviral agents in influenza: summary of Influenza Workshop VIII. J. infect. Dis. *134:* 516 (1976).

Coulon, P.; Rollin, P. E.; Flamand, A.: Molecular basis of rabies virus virulence. II. Identification of a site on the CVS glycoprotein associated with virulence. J. gen. Virol. *64:* 693 (1983).

Crumpacker, C. S.; Schnipper, L. E.; Marlowe, S. I.; Kowalsky, P. N.; Hershey, B. J.; Levin, M. J.: Resistance to antiviral drugs of herpes simplex virus isolated from a patient treated with acyclovir. New Engl. J. Med. *306:* 343 (1982).

Crumpton, M. J.: Protein antigens: the molecular basis of antigenicity and immunogenicity; in Sela, The antigens, vol. II (Academic Press, New York 1974).

Daemer, R. J.; Feinstone, S. M.; Gust, I. D.; Purcell, R. H.: Propagation of human hepatitis A virus in African green monkey cell culture: primary isolation and serila passage. Infect. Immunity *32:* 388 (1981).

Darby, G.; Field, H. J.; Salisbury, S. A.: Altered substrate specificity of herpes simplex virus thymidine kinase confers acyclovir-resistance. Nature, Lond. *289:* 81 (1981).

Davies, W. L.; Grunert, R. R.; Haff, R. F.; McGahen, J. W.; Neumayer, E. M.; Paulshock, M.; Watts, J. C.; Wood, T. R.; Hermann, E. C.; Hoffman, C. E.: Antiviral activity of 1-adamantanamine (Amantadine). Science *144:* 862 (1964).

Davis, A. R.; Bos, T.; Ueda, M.; Nayak, D. P.; Dowbenko, D.; Compans, R. W.: Immune response to human influenza virus hemagglutinin expressed in *Escherichia coli.* Gene *21:* 273 (1983).

de Clercq, E.: New trends in antiviral chemotherapy. Archs int. Physiol. Biochim. *87:* 353 (1979).

de Clercq, E.: Interferon inducers. Antibiot. Chemother. vol. 27, p. 251 (Karger, Basel 1980).

de Clercq, E.: Nucleoside analogues as antiviral agents. Acta microbiol. Acad. Sci. hung. *28:* 289 (1981).

de Clercq, E.: Specific targets for antiviral drugs. Biochem. J. *205:* 1 (1982a).

de Clercq, E.: BVDU [(*E*)-5-(2-bromovinyl)-2′-deoxyuridine]; in Becker, Antiviral drugs and interferon: molecular basis of their activity (Nijhoff, The Hague 1982b).

de Clercq, E.: Selective antiherpes agents. Trends pharmacol. Sci. *3:* 492 (1982c).

de Clercq, E.; Balzarini, J.; Descamps, J.; Huang, G.-F.; Torrence, P. F.; Bergstrom, D. E.; Jones, A. S.; Serafinowski, P.; Verhelst, G.; Walker, R. T.: Antiviral, antimetabolic, and cytotoxic activities of 5-substituted 2′-deoxycytidines. Molec. Pharmacol. *21:* 217 (1982).

de Clercq, E.; Degreef, H.; Wildiers, J.; deJonge, G.; Drochmans, A.; Deschamps, J.; deSomer, P.: Oral (*E*)-5-(2-bromovinyl)-2′-deoxyuridine in severe herpes zoster. Br. med. J. *281:* 1178 (1980a).

de Clercq, E.; Descamps, J.; deSomer, P.; Barr, P.J.; Jones, A.S.; Walker, R.T.: (*E*)-5-(2-bromovinyl)-2'-deoxyuridine: a potent and selective antiherpes agent. Proc. natn. Acad. Sci. USA *76:* 2947 (1979).

de Clercq, E.; Descamps, J.; Maudgal, P.C.; Missotten, L.; Leyten, R.; Verhelst, G.; Jones, A.S.; Walker, R.T.; Busson, R.; Vanderhaeghe, H.; deSomer, P.: Selective anti-herpes activity of 5-(2-halogenovinyl)-2'-deoxyuridines and -2'-deoxycytidines; in Collier, Oxford, Developments in antiviral therapy, pp. 21–42 (Academic Press, London 1980b).

de Clercq, E.; Descamps, J.; Verhelst, G.; Walker, R.T.; Jones, A.S.; Torrence, P.F.; Shugar, D.: Comparative efficacy of antiherpes drugs against different strains of herpes simplex virus. J. infect. Dis. *141:* 563 (1980c).

de Maeyer, E.; de Maeyer-Guignard, J.: Interferons. Compreh. Virol. *15:* 205 (1979).

de Maeyer, E.; de Maeyer-Guignard, J.: Immunoregulatory action of type I interferon in the mouse. Ann. N.Y Acad. Sci. *350:* 1 (1980).

de Maeyer, E.; Galasso, G.; Schellekens, H. (eds.): The biology of the interferon system (Elsevier/North-Holland, Amsterdam 1981).

de Maeyer, E.; Schellekens, H.: The biology of the interferon system 1983 (Elsevier, Amsterdam 1983).

Derynck, R.; Remaut, E.; Saman, E.; Stanssens, P.; de Clercq, E.; Content, J.; Fiers, W.: Expression of human fibroblast interferon gene in *Escherichia coli.* Nature, Lond. *287:* 193 (1980).

DeStefano, E.; Friedman, R.M.; Friedman-Kien, A.E.; Goedert, J.J.; Henricksen, D.; Preble, O.T.; Sonnabend, J.A.; Vilček, J.: Acid-labile human leukocyte interferon in homosexual men with Kaposi's sarcoma and lymphadenopathy. J. infect. Dis. *146;* 451 (1982).

de Weck, A.; Kristensen, F.; Landy, M. (eds.): Biochemical characterization of lymphokines (Academic Press, New York 1980).

Diana, G.D.; Salvador, U.J.; Zalay, E.S.; Carabateas, P.M.; Williams, G.L.; Collins, J.C.; Pancic, F.: Antiviral activity of some β-diketones. 2. Aryloxy alkyl diketones. In vitro activity against both RNA and DNA viruses. J. medicinal Chem. *20:* 757 (1977).

Dienstag, J.L.; Stevens, C.E.; Bahn, A.K.; Szmuness, W.: Hepatitis B vaccine administered to chronic carriers of hepatitis B surface antigen. Ann. intern. Med. *96:* 575 (1982).

Dietzschold, B.; Cohen, G.; Eisenberg, R.; Varrichio, A.: Synthesis of an antigenic determinant of the herpes simplex virus (HSV) glycoprotein D which stimulates the production of virus neutralizing antibodies and which confers protection against a lethal challenge infection of HSV; in Lerner; Chanock, Modern approaches to vaccines (Cold Spring Harbor Laboratory, New York 1984).

Doetsch, P.W.; Suhadolnik, R.J.; Sawada, Y.; Mosca, J.D.; Flick, M.B.; Reichenbach, N.L.; Dang, A.Q.; Wu, J.M.; Charubala, R.; Pfleiderer, W.; Henderson, E.E.: Core (2'-5') oligoadenylate and the cordycepin analog: inhibitors of Epstein-Barr virus-induced transformation of human lymphocytes in the absence of interferon. Proc. natn. Acad. Sci. USA *78:* 6699 (1981).

Dolin, R.; Reichman, R.C.; Madore, H.P.; Maynard, R.; Linton, P.N.; Webber-Jones, J.: A controlled trial of amantadine and rimantadine in the prophylaxis of influenza A infection. New Engl. J. med. *307:* 580 (1982).

Dowdle, W.R.: Influenza immunoprophylaxis after 30 years' experience; in Nayak, Genetic variation among influenza viruses; ICN-UCLA Symp., vol. 21, pp. 525–534 (Academic Press, New York 1981).

Dreesman, G. R.; Sanchez, Y.; Ionescu-Matiu, I.; Sparrow, J. T.; Six, H. R.; Peterson, D. L.; Hollinger, F. B.; Melnick, J. L.: Antibody to hepatitis B surface antigen after a single inoculation of uncoupled synthetic HBsAg peptides. Nature, Lond. *295:* 158 (1982).

Dubovi, E. J.; Geratz, J. D.; Shaver, S. R.; Tidwell, R. R.: Inhibition of respiratory syncytial virus-host cell interactions by mono- and diamidines. Antimicrob. Agents Chemother. *19:* 649 (1981).

Dudgeon, J. A.: Rubella: the U.K. experience. Dev. biol. Standard., vol. 43, p. 327 (Karger, Basel 1979).

Dunnick, J. K.; Galasso, G. J.: Clinical trials with exogenous interferon. J. infect. Dis. *139:* 109 (1979); *142:* 293 (1980).

Edelman, R.: Vaccine adjuvants. Rev. infect. Dis. *2:* 370 (1980).

Edelman, R.; Ascher, M. S.; Oster, C. N.; Ramsburg, H. H.; Cole, F. E.; Eddy, G. A.: Evaluation in humans of a new, inactivated vaccine for Venezuelan encephalitis virus (C-84). J. infect. Dis. *140:* 708 (1979).

Edelman, R.; Hardegree, M. C.; Chedid, L.: Summary of an international symposium on potentiation of the immune response to vaccines. J. infect. Dis. *141:* 103 (1980).

Edge, M. D.; Greene, A. R.; Heathcliffe, G. R.; Meacock, P. A.; Schuch, W.; Scanlon, D. B.; Atkinson, T. C.; Newton, C. R.; Markham, A. F.: Total synthesis of a human leukocyte interferon gene. Nature, Lond. *292:* 756 (1981).

Edman, J. C.; Hallewell, R. A.; Valenzuela, P.; Goodman, H. M.; Rutter, W. J.: Synthesis of hepatitis B surface and core antigens in *E. coli.* Nature, Lond. *291:* 503 (1981).

Edy, V. G.; Augenstein, D. C.; Edwards, C. R.; Cruttenden, V. F.; Lubinecki, A. S.: Large-scale tissue culture for human IFN-β production. Tex. Rep. Biol. Med. *41:* 169 (1982).

Eggers, H. J.: Successful treatment of enterovirus-infected mice by 2-(α-hydroxybenzyl)-benzimidazole and guanidine. J. exp. Med. *143:* 1367 (1976).

Elek, S. D.; Stern, H.: Development of a vaccine against mental retardation caused by cytomegalovirus infection *in utero.* Lancet *i:* 1 (1974).

Elion, G. B.: The chemotherapeutic exploitation of virus-specified enzymes. Adv. Enzyme Reguln *18:* 53 (1980).

Elion, G. B.; Furman, P. A.; Fyfe, J. A.; deMiranda, P.; Beauchamp, L.; Schaeffer, H. J.: Selectivity of action of an antiherpetic agent, 9-(2-hydroxyethoxymethyl) guanine. Proc. natn. Acad. Sci. USA *74:* 5716 (1977).

Emini, E. A.; Jameson, B. A.; Wimmer, E.: Priming for and induction of anti-poliovirus neutralizing antibodies by synthetic peptides. Nature, Lond. *304:* 699 (1983).

Emtage, J. S.; Carey, N. H.: The production of vaccines by recombinant DNA techniques; in New developments with human and veterinary vaccines. Progr. clin. biol. Res. *47:* 367 (Liss, New York 1980).

Emtage, J. S.; Tacon, W. C. A.; Catlin, G. H.; Jenkins, B.; Porter, A. G.; Carey, N. H.: Influenza antigenic determinants are expressed from haemagglutinin genes cloned in *Escherichia coli.* Nature, Lond. *283:* 171 (1980).

Epstein, M. A.; Achong, B. G.: The Epstein-Barr virus (Springer, Berlin 1979).

Epstein, L. B.: Interferon-gamma: is it really different from other interferons? in Gresser, Interferon 3, pp. 13–44 (Academic Press, New York 1981).

Epstein, M. A.; North, J. R.; Morgan, A. J.: Possibilities for antiviral vaccine intervention in nasopharyngeal carcinoma; in Proc. 3rd Int. Symp. on Nasopharyngeal Carcinoma (1983).

Eriksson, B.; Helgstrand, E.; Johansson, N.G.; Larsson, A.; Misiorny, A.; Noren, J.O.; Philipson, L.; Stenberg, K.; Stening, G.; Stridh, S.; Öberg, B.: Inhibition of influenza virus ribonucleic acid polymerase by ribavirin triphosphate. Antimicrob. Agents Chemother. *11:* 946 (1977).

Farrell, P.J.; Sen, G.C.; Dubois, M.F.; Ratner, L.; Slattery, E.; Lengyel, P.: Interferon action: two distinct pathways for inhibition of protein synthesis by double-stranded RNA. Proc. natn. Acad. Sci. USA *75:* 5893 (1978).

Feldmann, M.; Schreier, M. (ed.): Lymphokines 5. Monoclonal T cells and their products (Academic Press, New York 1982).

Fenner, F.: The possible use of temperature-sensitive conditional lethal mutants for immunization in viral infections; in Kohn, Klinberg, Immunity in viral and rickettsial diseases, p. 131 (Plenum Press, New York 1972).

Fenner, F.: A successful eradication campaign. Global eradication of smallpox. Rev. infect. Dis. *4:* 916 (1982).

Fiddian, A.P.; Yeo, J.M.; Stubbings, R.; Dean, D.: Successful treatment of herpes labialis with topical acyclovir. Br. med. J. *286:* 1699 (1983).

Field, H.J.; McMilan, A.; Darby, G.: The sensitivity of acyclovir-resistant mutants of herpes simplex virus to other antiviral drugs. J. infect. Dis. *143:* 281 (1981).

Field, H.J.; Phillips, I. (eds.): Acyclovir. J. antimicrob. Chemother., vol. *12:* suppl. B (Academic Press, London 1983).

Field, H.J.; Wildy, P.: The pathogenicity of thymidine kinase-deficient mutants of herpes simplex virus in mice. J. Hyg., Camb. *81:* 267 (1978).

Finter, N.B.: Large-scale production of human interferon from lymphoblastoid cells. Tex. Rep. Biol. Med. *41:* 175 (1982).

Finter, N.B.; Billiau, A.; Friedman, R.; Vilček, J.; de Maeyer, E.: Interferons; 3rd ed., vol. 1–4 (Elsevier/North-Holland, Amsterdam 1984).

Fleischmann, W.R.: Potentiation of the direct anticellular activity of mouse interferons: mutual synergism and interferon concentration dependence. Cancer Res. *42:* 869 (1982).

Fox, J.P.; Hall, C.E.: Viruses in families (PSG Publ., Littleton, Mass. 1980).

Fox, J.S.; White, D.O.: Delivery of antiviral chemotherapeutic agents to neurons by retrograde axonal transport. Med. Hypotheses *6:* 773 (1980).

Friedman, R.M.: Antiviral activity of interferons. Bact. Rev. *41:* 543 (1977).

Friedman, R.M.: Interferons: a primer (Academic Press, New York 1981).

Furman, P.A.; Coen, D.M.; St. Clair, M.H.; Schaffer, P.A.: Acyclovir-resistant mutants of herpes simplex virus type 1 express altered DNA polymerase or reduced acyclovir phosphorylating activities. J. Virol. *40:* 936 (1981).

Galasso, G.J.: An assessment of antiviral drugs for the management of infectious diseases in humans. Antiviral Res. *1:* 73 (1981a).

Galasso, G.J.: Antiviral agents for the control of viral diseases. Bull. Wld Hlth Org. *59:* 503 (1981b).

Galasso, G.J.; Merigan, T.C.; Buchanan, R.A. (eds.): Antiviral agents and viral diseases of man (Raven Press, New York 1979).

Gandhi, S.S.; Stanley, P.M.; Taylor, J.M.; White, D.O.: Inhibition of influenza viral glycoprotein synthesis by sugars. Microbios *5:* 41 (1972).

Gauri, K. K. (ed.): Antiviral chemotherapy: design of inhibitors of viral functions (Academic Press, New York 1981).

Gerin, J. L.; Alexander, H.; Shih, J. W. K.; Purcell, R. H.; Dapolito, G.; Engle, R.; Green, N.; Sutcliffe, J. G.; Shinnick, T. M.; Lerner, R. A.: Chemically synthesized peptides of hepatitis B surface antigen duplicate the *d/y* specificities and induce subtype-specific antibodies in chimpanzees. Proc. natn. Acad. Sci. USA *80:* 2365 (1983).

Gershon, A. A.: Live attenuated varicella-zoster vaccine. Rev. infect. Dis. *2:* 393 (1980).

Gething, M.-J.; Sambrook, J.: Cell-surface expression of influenza haemagglutinin from a cloned DNA copy of the RNA gene. Nature, Lond. *293:* 620 (1981).

Gidlund, M.; Örn, A.; Wigzell, H.; Senik, A.; Gresser, I.: Enhanced NK cell activity in mice injected with interferon and interferon inducers. Nature, Lond. *223:* 259 (1978).

Goeddel, D. V.; Leung, D. W.; Dull, T. J.; Gross, M.; Lawn, R. M.; McCandliss, R.; Seeburg, P. H.; Ullrich, A.; Yelverton, E.; Gray, P. W.: The structure of eight distinct cloned human leukocyte interferon cDNAs. Nature, Lond. *290:* 20 (1981).

Goeddel, D. V.; Shepard, H. M.; Yelverton, E.; Leung, D.; Crea, R.; Sloma, A.; Pestka, S.: Synthesis of human fibroblast interferon by *E. coli.* Nucl. Acids Res. *8:* 4057 (1980a).

Goeddel, D. V.; Yelverton, E.; Ullrich, A.; Heyneker, H. L.; Miozzari, G.; Holmes, W.; Seeburg, P. H.; Dull, T.; May, L.; Stebbing, N.; Crea, R.; Maeda, S.; McCandliss, R.; Sloma, A.; Tabor, J. M.; Gross, M.; Familletti, P. C.; Pestka, S.: Human leukocyte interferon produced by *E. coli* is biologically active. Nature, Lond. *287:* 411 (1980b).

Gordon, J.; Minks, M. A.: The interferon renaissance: molecular aspects of induction and action. Microbiol. Rev. *45:* 244 (1981).

Gray, P. W.; Goeddel, D. V.: Structure of the human immune interferon gene. Nature, Lond. *298:* 859 (1982).

Gray, P. W.; Leung, D. W.; Pennica, D.; Yelverton, E.; Najarian, R.; Simonsen, C. C.; Derynck, R.; Sherwood, P. J.; Wallace, D. M.; Berger, S. L.; Levinson, A. D.; Goeddel, D. V.: Expression of human immune interferon cDNA in *E. coli* and monkey cells. Nature, Lond. *295:* 503 (1982).

Green, N.; Alexander, H.; Olson, A.; Alexander, S.; Shinnick, T. M.; Sutcliffe, J. G.; Lerner, R. A.: Immunogenic structure of the influenza virus hemagglutinin. Cell *28:* 477 (1982).

Greenberg, S. B.; Harmon, M. W.; Couch, R. B.; Johnson, P. E.; Wilson, S. Z.; Dacso, C. C.; Bloom, K.; Quarles, J.: Prophylactic effect of low doses of human leukocyte interferon against infection with rhinovirus. J. infect. Dis. *145:* 542 (1982).

Gregoriadis, G.: The carrier potential of liposomes in biology and medicine. New Engl. J. Med. *295:* 704–710, 765–770 (1976).

Gregoriadis, G.: Targeting of drugs: possibilities in viral chemotherapy and prophylaxis. Pharmacol. Ther. *10:* 103 (1980).

Gresser, I.: On the varied biological effects of interferon. Cell. Immunol. *34:* 406 (1977).

Gresser, I. (ed.): Interferon 1, 2, 3, 4 (Academic Press, New York 1979, 1980, 1981, 1982).

Gresser, I., de Maeyer-Guignard, J.; Tovey, M. G.; de Maeyer, E.: Electrophoretically pure mouse interferon exerts multiple biologic effects. Proc. natn. Acad. Sci USA *76:* 5308 (1979).

Gresser, I.; Tovey, M. G.: Antitumor effects of interferon. Biochim. biophys. Acta *516:* 231 (1978).

Grundy, J. E.; Trapman, J.; Allan, J. E.; Shellam, G. R.; Melief, C. J. M.: Evidence for a protective role of interferon in resistance to murine cytomegalovirus and its control by non-H2-linked genes. Infect. Immunity *37:* 143 (1982).

Grunert, R.R.: Search for antiviral agents. A. Rev. Microbiol. *33:* 335 (1979).

Gutterman, J.U.; Blumenschein, G.R.; Alexanian, R.; Yap, H.-Y.; Buzdar, A.U.; Cabanillas, F.; Hortobagyi, G.N.; Hersh, E.M.; Rasmussen, S.L.; Harmon, M.; Kramer, M.; Pestka, S.: Leukocyte interferon-induced tumor regression in human metastatic breast cancer, multiple myeloma, and malignant lymphoma. Ann. intern. Med. *93:* 399 (1980).

Gutterman, J.U.; Fine, S.; Quesaday, J.; Horning, S.J.; Levine, J.F.; Alexanian, R.; Bernhardt, L.; Kramer, M.; Spiegel, H.; Colburn, W.; Trown, P.; Merigan, T.C.; Dziewanowski, Z.: Recombinant human leukocyte A interferon: pharmacokinetics single-dose tolerance, and biologic effects in cancer patients. Ann. intern. Med. *96:* 549 (1982).

Hackett, C.J.; Dietzschold, B.; Gerhard, W.; Ghrist, B.; Knorr, R.; Gillissen, D.; Melchers, F.: The influenza virus site recognized by a murine helper T cell specific for H1 strains: localization of a nine amino acid sequence in the hemagglutinin molecule. J. exp. Med. *158:* 294 (1983).

Hahn, F.E. (ed.): Virus chemotherapy. Antibiot. Chemother., vol. 27 (Karger, Basel 1980).

Hall, C.B.: Prevention of infections with respiratory syncytial virus: the hopes and hurdles ahead. Rev. infect. Dis. *2:* 384 (1980).

Hall, C.B.; McBride, J T.; Walsh, E.E.; Bell, D.M.; Gala, C.L.; Hildreth, S.; Ten Eyck, L.G.; Hall, W. J.: Aerosolized ribavirin treatment of infants with respiratory syncytial viral infection. New Engl. J. Med. *308:* 1443 (1983).

Haller, O.; Arnheiter, H.; Gresser, I.; Lindenmann, J.: Virus-specific interferon action: protection of newborn Mx carriers against lethal infection with influenza virus. J. exp. Med. *154:* 199 (1981).

Haller, O.; Arnheiter, H.; Horisberger, M.A.; Gresser, I.; Lindenmann, J.: Interaction between interferon and host genes in antiviral defense. Ann. N.Y. Acad. Sci. *350:* 558 (1980).

Halstead, S.B.: The pathogenesis of dengue. Molecular epidemiology in infectious disease. Am. J. Epidem. *114:* 632 (1981).

Hammon, W. McD.; Kitaoka, M.; Downs, W.G.: Immunization for Japanese encephalitis (Igaku Shoin, Tokyo 1971).

Hay, A.J.; Kennedy, N.C.T.; Skehel, J.J.; Appleyard, G.: The matrix protein gene determined amantadine-sensitivity of influenza viruses. J. gen. Virol. *42:* 189 (1979).

Hayden, F.G.; Gwaltney, J.M.: Prophylactic activity of intranasal enviroxime against experimentally induced rhinovirus type 39 infection. Antimicrob. Agents Chemother. *21:* 892 (1982).

Hayden, G.F.; Preblud, S.R.; Orenstein, W.A.; Conrad, J.L.: The current status of mumps and mumps vaccine in the United States. Pediatrics, Springfield *62:* 965 (1978).

Helenius, A.; Kartenbeck, J.; Simons, K.; Fries, E.: On the entry of Semliki Forest virus into BHK-21 cells. J. Cell Biol. *84:* 404 (1980).

Helgstrand, E.; Flodh, H.; Lernestedt, J.-O.; Lundstrom, J.; Oberg, B.: Trisodium phosphonoformate: antiviral activities, safety evaluation and preliminary clinical results; in Collier, Oxford, Developments in antiviral therapy, pp. 63–83 (Academic Press, London 1980).

Hennessen, W.; van Wezel, A.L. (eds.): Reassessment of inactivated poliomyelitis vaccine. Dev. biol. Standard., vol. 47 (Karger, Basel 1981).

Herrmann, E. C.: Plaque inhibition test for detection of specific inhibitors of DNA containing viruses. Proc. Soc. exp. Biol. Med. *107:* 142 (1961).

Herrmann, E. C. (ed.): Third conference on antiviral substances. Ann. N.Y. Acad. Sci. *284:* 1–720 (1977).

Hill, J. M.; Gangarosa, L. P.; Park, N. H.: Iontophoretic application of antiviral chemotherapeutic agents. Ann. N.Y. Acad. Sci. *284:* 604 (1977).

Hilleman, M. R.: New developments with new vaccines; in Mizrahi et al., New developments with human and veterinary vaccines. Prog. clin. biol. Res. *47:* 21 (Liss, New York 1980).

Hilleman, M. R.; Buynak, E. B.; McAleer, W. J.; McLean, A. A.; Provost, P. J.; Tytell, A. A.: Newer developments with human hepatitis vaccines. Perspect. Virol. *11:* 219 (1981a).

Hilleman, M. R.; Buynak, E. B.; McAleer, W. J.; McLean, A. A.; Provost, P. J.; Tytell, A. A.: Hepatitis A and hepatitis B vaccines; in Szmuness, Alter, Maynard, Viral hepatitis, pp. 385–397 (Franklin Institute Press, Philadelphia 1982).

Hilleman, M. R.; Larson, V. M.; Lehman, E. D.; Salerno, R. A.; Conrad, R. G.; McLean, A. A.: Subunit herpes simplex 2 vaccine; in Nahmias, Dowdle, Schinazi, The human herpesviruses, pp. 503–506 (Elsevier, New York 1981).

Hinman, A. R.; Brandling-Bennett, A. D.; Bernier, R. H.; Kirby, C. D.; Eddins, D. L.: Current features of measles in the United States: feasibility of meales elimination. Epidemiol. Rev. *2:* 153 (1980).

Hirsch, M. S.; Swartz, M. N.: Antiviral agents. New Engl. J. Med. *302:* 903–907, 949–953 (1980).

Hirsch, M. S.; Schooley, R. T.; Cosimi, A. B.; Russell, P. S.; Delmonico, F. L.; Tolkoff-Rubin, N. E.; Herrin, J. T.; Cantell, K.; Farrell, M.-L.; Rota, T. R.; Rubin, R. H.: Effects of interferon-alpha on cytomegalovirus reactivation syndromes in renal transplant recipients. New Engl. J. Med. *308:* 1489 (1983).

Hitzeman, R. A.; Hagie, F. E.; Levine, H. L.; Goeddel, D. V.; Ammerer, G.; Hall, B. D.: Expression of a human gene for interferon in yeast. Nature, Lond. *293:* 717 (1981).

Hollinger, F. B.; Adam, E.; Heiberg, D.; Melnick, J. L.: Response to hepatitis B vaccine in a young adult population; in Szmuness, Alter, Maynard, Viral hepatitis, pp. 361–372 (Franklin Institute Press, Philadelphia 1982).

Horstmann, D. M.: Viral vaccines and their ways. Rev. infect. Dis. *1:* 502 (1979).

Hoskins, T. W.; Davies, J. R.; Smith, A. J.; Miller, C. L.; Allchin, A.: Assessment of inactivated influenza-A vaccine after three outbreaks of influenza A at Christ's Hospital. Lancet *i:* 33 (1979).

Hovanessian, A. G.; la Bonnardiere, C.; Falcoff, E.: Action of murine γ (immune) interferon on β (fibroblast)-interferon resistant L1210 and embryonal carcinoma cells. J. Interferon Res. *1:* 125 (1980).

Ikič, D.; Nola, P.; Maricic, Z.; Smudj, K.; Oresic, V.; Knezevic, M.; Rode, B.; Jusic, D.; Soos, E.: Application of human leukocyte interferon in patients with urinary bladder papillomatosis, breast cancer and melanoma. Lancet *i:* 1022 (1981).

Ionescu-Matiu, I.; Kennedy, R. C.; Sparrow, J. T.; Culwell, A. R.; Sanchez, Y.; Melnick, J. L.; Dreesman, G. R.: Epitopes associated with a synthetic hepatitis B surface antigen peptide. J. Immun. *130:* 1947 (1983).

Isaacs, A.; Lindenmann, J.: Virus interference. I. The interferon. Proc. R. Soc., Lond. B *147:* 258 (1957).

Ishitsuka, H.; Ninomiya, Y.T.; Ohsawa, C.; Fujiu, M.; Suhara, Y.: Direct and specific inactivation of rhinovirus by chalcone Ro 09-0410. Antimicrob. Agents Chemother. *22:* 617 (1982).

Jackson, D.C.; Murray, J.M.; Brown, L.E.; White, D.O.: Immunological properties of influenza virus hemagglutinin and its fragments; in Nayak, Genetic variation among influenza viruses; ICN-UCLA Symp., vol. 21, pp. 547–566 (Academic Press, New York 1981).

Jackson, D.C.; Murray, J.M.; White, D.O.; Fagan, C.N.; Tregear, G.W.: Antigenic activity of a synthetic peptide comprising the 'loop' region of influenza virus hemagglutinin. Virology *120:* 273 (1982).

Jacobs, L.; O'Malley, J.; Freeman, A.; Ekes, R.: Intrathecal interferon reduces exacerbations of multiple sclerosis. Science *214:* 1026 (1981).

Jahrling, P.B.; Hesse, R.A.; Eddy, G.A.; Johnson, K.M.; Callis, R.T.; Stephen, E.L.: Lassa virus infection of rhesus monkeys: pathogenesis and treatment with ribavirin. J. infect. Dis. *141:* 580 (1980).

Johnson, H.M.; Baron, S.: Evaluation of effects of interferon and interferon inducers on the immune response. Pharmacol. Ther. A *1:* 349 (1977).

Jones, B.R.; Coster, D.J.; Fison, P.N.; Thompson, G.M.; Cobo, L.M.; Falcon, M.G.: Efficacy of acycloguanosine (Wellcome 248U) against herpes-simplex corneal ulcers. Lancet *i:* 243 (1979).

Juel-Jensen, B.E.: Results of the treatment of zoster with idoxuridine in dimethyl sulfoxide. Ann. N.Y. Acad. Sci. *173:* 74 (1970).

Kadish, A.S.; Tarsey, F.A.; Yu, G.S.M.; Doyle, A.T.; Bloom, B.R.: Interferon as a mediator of human lymphocyte suppression. J. exp. Med. *151:* 637 (1980).

Kaufman, H.E.: Clinical cure of herpes simplex keratitis by 5-iodo-2′-deoxyuridine. Proc. Soc. exp. Biol. Med. *109:* 251 (1962).

Kendal, A.P.; Maassab, H.F.; Alexandrova, G.I.; Ghendon, Y.Z.: Development of cold-adapted recombinant live attenuated influenza A vaccines in the US and USSR. Antiviral Res. *1:* 339 (1982).

Kerr, I.M.; Brown, R.E.: pppA2′p5′A2′p5′A: an inhibitor of protein synthesis synthesized with an enzyme fraction from interferon-treated cells. Proc. natn. Acad. Sci. USA *75:* 256 (1978).

Kerr, I.M.; Brown, R.E.; Ball, L.A.: Increased sensitivity of cell-free protein synthesis to double-stranded RNA after interferon treatment. Nature, Lond. *250:* 57 (1974).

Kew, O.M.; Nottay, B.K.; Hatch, M.H.; Nakano, J.H.; Obijeski, J.F.: Multiple genetic changes in the oral poliovaccines upon replication in humans. J. gen. Virol. *56:* 337 (1981).

Kimchi, A.; Shure, H.; Revel, M.: Anti-mitogenic function of interferon-induced (2′5′) oligoadenylate and growth-related variations in enzymes that synthesize and degrade this oligonucleotide. Eur. J. Biochem. *114:* 5 (1981).

King, D.H.; Galasso, G. (eds.): Proceedings of a symposium on Acyclovir. Am. J. Med. *73:* 1–393 (1982).

Kitamura, N.; Semler, B.L.; Rothberg, P.G.; Larsen, G.R.; Adler, C.J.; Dorner, A.J.; Emini, E.A.; Hanecak, R.; Lee, J.J.; van der Werf, S.; Anderson, C.W.; Wimmer, E.: Primary structure, gene organization and polypeptide expression of poliovirus RNA. Nature, Lond. *291:* 547 (1981).

Kleid, D.G.; Yansura, D.; Small, B.; Dowbenko, D.; Moore, D.M.; Grubman, M.J.;

McKercher, P. D.; Morgan, D. O.; Robertson, B. H.; Bachrach, H. L.: Cloned viral protein vaccine for foot-and-mouth disease: responses in cattle and swine. Science *214:* 1125 (1981).

Klenk, H.-D.; Schwarz, R. T.: Viral glycoprotein metabolism as a target for antiviral substances. Antiviral Res. *2:* 177 (1982).

Knight, E.; Fahey, D.: Human fibroblast interferon. An improved purification. J. biol. Chem. *256:* 3609 (1981).

Knight, V.; McClung, H. W.; Wilson, S. Z.; Waters, B. K.; Quarles, J. M.; Cameron, R. W.; Greggs, S. E.; Zerwas, J. M.; Couch, R. B.: Ribavirin small-particle aerosol treatment of influenza. Lancet *ii:* 945 (1981).

Knight, V.; Wilson, S. Z.; Wyde, P. R.; Drake, S.; Couch, R. B.; Galegov, G. A.; Novokhatska, A. S.: Small particle aerosols of amantadine and ribavirin in the treatment of influenza; in Smith, Kirkpatrick, Ribavirin, pp. 129–146 (Academic Press, New York 1980).

Knop, J.; Stemmer, R.; Neumann, C.; de Maeyer, E.; Macher, E.: Interferon inhibits the suppressor T cell response of delayed-type hypersensitivity. Nature, Lond. *296:* 757 (1982).

Knox, E. G.: Strategy for rubella vaccination. Int. J. Epidem. *9:* 13 (1980).

Kono, R. (ed.): Proc. Conf. on Clinical Potential of Interferon in Viral Diseases and Malignant Tumours (Tokyo University Press, Tokyo 1982).

Korant, B. D.: in Gauri, Antiviral chemotherapy: design of inhibitors of viral functions, pp. 37–47 (Academic Press, New York 1981).

Korant, B. D.; Chow, N. L.; Lively, M. O.; Powers, J. C.: Proteolytic events in replication of animal viruses. Ann. N.Y. Acad. Sci. *343:* 304 (1980).

Krugman, S.: Present status of measles and rubella immunization in the United States: a medical progress report. J. Pediat. *90:* 1 (1977).

Küpper, H.; Keller, W.; Kurz, C.; Forss, S.; Schaller, H.; Franze, R.; Strohmaier, K.; Marquardt, O.; Zaslavsky, V. G.; Hofschneider, P. H.: Cloning of cDNA of major antigen of foot and mouth disease virus and expression in *E. coli.* Nature, Lond. *289:* 555 (1981).

Lai, C.-J.; Markoff, L. J.; Zimmerman, S.; Cohen, B.; Berdt, J. A.; Chanock, R. M.: Cloning DNA sequences from influenza viral RNA segments. Proc. natn. Acad. Sci. USA *77:* 210 (1980).

Lamb, J. R.; Eckels, D. D.; Lake, P.; Woody, J. N.; Green, N.: Human T cell clones recognizing chemically synthesized peptides of influenza haemagglutinin. Nature, Lond. *300:* 66 (1982).

Lampson, G. P.; Field, A. K.; Tytell, A. A.; Hilleman, M. R.: PolyI:C/poly-*L*-lysine: potent inducer of interferons in primates. J. Interferon Res. *1:* 539 (1982).

Lang, D. J.; Cytomegalovirus immunization: status, prospects and problems. Rev. infect. Dis. *2:* 449 (1980).

Larnicol, N.; Augery, Y.; le Bousse-Kerdiles, C.; Degiorgis, V.; Chermann, J. C.; Teze, A.; Jasmin, C.: In vivo effect of a new mineral condensed ion (HPA 39) on murine Friend leukaemia. J. gen. Virol. *55:* 17 (1981).

Laver, W. G.; Air, G. M. (eds.): Structure and variation in influenza virus (Elsevier/North-Holland, Amsterdam 1980).

Lebleu, B.; Content, J.: Mechanisms of interferon action: biochemical and genetic approaches; in Gresser, Interferon 4, pp. 47–94 (Academic Press, London 1982).

Lebleu, B.; Sen, G.C.; Shaila, S.; Cabrer, B.; Lengyel, P.: Interferon, double-stranded RNA and protein phosphorylation. Proc. natn. Acad. Sci. USA *73:* 3107 (1976).

Lee, S.H.; Weck, P.K.; Moore, J.; Chen, S.; Stebbing, N.: Pharmacological comparison of two hybrid recombinant DNA-derived human leukocyte interferons; in Merigan, Friedman, Interferons, UCLA Symp. on Mol. Cell. Biology, vol. XXV, pp. 341–352 (Academic Press, New York 1982).

Lengyel, P.: Mechanisms of interferon action: the (2′-5′) $(A)_n$ synthetase-RNase L pathway; in Gresser, Interferon 3, pp. 77–99 (Academic Press, New York 1981).

Lengyel, P.: Biochemistry of interferons and their actions. A. Rev. Biochem. *51:* 251 (1982).

Leong, S.S.; Horoszewicz, J.S.: Production and preparation of human fibroblast interferon for clinical trials. Meth. Enzym. *78:* 87 (1981).

Lerner, R.A.: Tapping the immunological repertoire to produce antibodies of predetermined specificity. Nature, Lond. *299:* 592 (1982).

Lerner, R.A.; Chanock, R.M. (eds.): Modern approaches to vaccines (Cold Spring Harbor Laboratory, New York 1984).

Lerner, R.A.; Green, R.A.; Alexander, H.; Liu, F.T.; Sutcliffe, J.G.; Shinnick, T.M.: Chemically synthesized peptides predicted from the nucleotide sequence of the hepatitis B virus genome elicit antibodies reactive with native envelope protein of Dane particles. Proc. natn. Acad. Sci. USA *78:* 3403 (1981).

Levandowski, R.A.; Pachucki, C.T.; Rubenis, M.; Jackson, G.G.: Topical enviroxime against rhinovirus infection. Antimicrob. Agents Chemother. *22:* 1004 (1982).

Levine, A.S.; Sivulich, M.; Wiernik, P.H.; Levy, H.B.: Initial clinical trials in cancer patients of polyriboinosinic-polyribocytidylic acid stabilized with poly-*L*-lysine, in carboxymethylcellulose [poly(ICLC)], a highly effective interferon inducer. Cancer Res. *39:* 1645 (1979).

Levy, W.P.; Rubinstein, M.; Shively, J.; del Valle, U.; Lai, C.-Y.; Moschera, J.; Brink, L.; Gerber, L.; Stein, S.; Pestka, S.: Amino acid sequence of a human leukocyte interferon. Proc. natn. Acad. Sci. USA *78:* 6186 (1981).

Lindahl, P.; Leary, P.; Gresser, I.: Enhancement by interferon of the specific toxicity of sensitized lymphocytes. Proc. natn. Acad. Sci. USA *69:* 721 (1972).

Lubeck, M.D.; Schulman, J.L.; Palese, P.: Susceptibility of influenza A viruses to amantadine is influenced by the gene coding for M protein. J. Virol. *28:* 710 (1978).

Maassab, H.F.; Monto, A.S.; deBorde, D.C.; Cox, N.J.; Kendal, A.P.: Development of cold recombinants of influenza virus as live virus vaccines; in Nayak, Genetic variation among influenza viruses. ICN-UCLA Symp., vol. 21, pp. 617–637 (Academic Press, New York 1981).

McAleer, W.J.; Markus, H.Z.; McLean, A.A.; Buynak, E.B.; Hilleman, M.R.: Stability on storage at various temperatures of live measles, mumps and rubella virus vaccines in new stabilizer. J. biol. Stand. *8:* 281 (1980).

Machida, H.; Kuninaka, A.; Yoshino, H.: Inhibitory effects of antiherpesviral thymidine analogs against varicella-zoster virus. Antimicrob. Agents Chemother. *21:* 358 (1982).

Mackay, P.; Pasek, M.; Magazin, M.; Kovacic, R.T.; Allet, B.; Stahl, S.; Gilbert, W.; Schaller, H.; Bruce, S.A.; Murray, K.: Production of immunologically active surface antigens of hepatitis B virus by *Escherichia coli.* Proc. natn. Acad. Sci. USA *78:* 4510 (1981).

McKinlay, M. A.; Miralles, J. V.; Brisson, C. J.; Pancic, F.: Prevention of human poliovirus-induced paralysis and death in mice by the novel antiviral agent arildone. Antimicrob. Agents Chemother. *22:* 1022 (1982).

McSharry, J. J.; Caliguiri, L. A.; Eggers, H. J.: Inhibition of uncoating of polioviruses by arildone, a new antiviral drug. Virology *97:* 307 (1979).

Maniatis, T.; Frisch, E. F.; Sambrook, J.: Molecular cloning: a laboratory manual (Cold Spring Harbor Laboratory, New York 1982).

Mantei, N.; Weissmann, C.: Controlled transcription of a human α-interferon gene introduced into mouse L cells. Nature, Lond. *297:* 128 (1982).

Marcus, P. I.: The interferon inducer moiety of viruses: a single molecule of dsRNA. Tex. Rep. Biol. Med. *41:* 70 (1982).

Maupas, P.; Goudeau, A.; Coursaget, P.; Drucker, J.; Bagros, P.: Immunization against hepatitis B in man. Lancet *i:* 1367 (1976).

Maupas, P.; Guesry, P. (eds.): Hepatitis B vaccine. Inserm Symp., vol. 18 (Elsevier/North-Holland, Amsterdam 1981).

Melnick, J. L.: Viral vaccines. Prog. med. Virol., vol. 23, p. 158 (Karger, Basel 1977).

Melnick, J. L.: Advantages and disadvantages of killed and live poliomyelitis vaccines. Bull. Wld Hlth Org. *56:* 21 (1978).

Melnick, J. L.: Poliomyelitis vaccines: an appraisal after 25 years. Compr. Ther. *6:* 6 (1980).

Merigan, T. C.: Antivirals with clinical potential. J. infect. Dis. *133:* suppl., pp. A1–A285 (1976).

Merigan, T. C.: Present appraisal of and future hopes for clinical utilization of human interferons; in Gresser, Interferon 3, pp. 135–154 (Academic Press, New York 1981a).

Merigan, T. C.: Chemotherapy for viral diseases. Perspect. Virol. *11:* 249 (1981b).

Merigan, T. C.; Friedman, R. M.: Interferons. UCLA Symp. on Mol. Cell. Biology, vol. XXV (Academic Press, New York 1982).

Merigan, T. C.; Reed, S. E.; Hall, T. S.; Tyrrell, D. A. J.: Inhibition of respiratory virus infection by locally applied interferon. Lancet *i:* 563 (1973).

Merz, D. C.; Scheid, A.; Choppin, P. W.: Importance of antibodies to the fusion glycoprotein of paramyxoviruses in the prevention of spread of infection. J. exp. Med. *151:* 275 (1980).

Meyer, H. M.; Hopps, H. E.; Parkman, P. D.: Appraisal and reappraisal of viral vaccines. Adv. intern. Med. *25:* 533 (1980).

Miller, D. L.; Kung, H.-F.; Pestka, S.: Crystallization of recombinant human leukocyte interferon A. Science *215:* 689 (1982).

Mims, C. A.; White, D. O.: Viral pathogenesis and immunology (Blackwell, Oxford 1984).

Mindel, A.; Adler, M. W.; Sutherland, S.; Fiddian, A. P.: Intravenous acyclovir treatment for primary genital herpes. Lancet *i:* 697 (1982).

Mitchell, C. D.; Bean, B.; Gentry, S. R.; Groth, K. E.; Boen, J. R.; Balfour, H. H.: Acyclovir therapy for mucocutaneous herpes simplex infections in immunocompromised patients. Lancet *i:* 1389 (1981).

Miyanohara, A.; Toh-e, A.; Nozaki, C.; Hamada, F.; Ohtomo, N.; Matsubara, K.: Expression of hepatitis B surface antigen in yeast. Proc. natn. Acad. Sci. USA *80:* 1 (1983).

Möller, G. (ed.): Antibody carriers of drugs and toxins in tumor therapy. Immunol. Rev. *62:* (1982a).

Möller, G. (ed.): Interleukins and lymphocyte activation. Immunol. Rev. *63:* (1982b).

Monath, T.P.; Kinney, R.M.; Schlesinger, J.J.; Brandriss, M.W.; Bres, P.: Ontogeny of yellow fever 17D vaccine: RNA oligonucleotide fingerprint and monoclonal antibody analysis of vaccines produced world-wide. J. gen. Virol. *64:* 627 (1983).

Montagnon, B.J.; Janget, B.; Nicolas, A.J.: The large scale cultivation of VERO cells in micjrocarrier culture for virus vaccine production. Preliminary results for killed poliovirus vaccine. Dev. biol. Standard., vol. 47, p. 55 (Karger, Basel 1981).

Moore, M.; Katona, P.; Kaplan, J.E.; Schonberger, L.B.; Hatch, M.H.: Poliomyelitis in the United States, 1969–1981. J. infect. Dis. *146:* 558 (1982).

Morley, D.C.: Severe measles: a barometer of childhood nutrition; in André, Potency and efficacy of vaccines, pp. 143–156 (Smith Kline-RIT, USA 1980).

Mozes, L.W.; Schultz, J.; Scott, W.A.; Werner, R. (eds.): Cellular responses to molecular modulators. Miami Winter Symp., vol. 18 (Academic Press, New York 1981).

Müller, G.M.; Shapira, M.; Arnon, R.: Anti-influenza response achieved by immunization with a synthetic conjugate. Proc. natn. Acad. Sci. USA *79:* 569 (1982).

Müller, W.E.G.: Mechanisms of action and pharmacology: chemical agents; in Galasso, Merigan, Buchanan, Antiviral agents and viral diseases of man, pp. 77–149 (Raven Press, New York 1979).

Munk, K.; Kirchner, H.: Interferons: properties, mode of action, production, clinical application (Karger, Basel 1982).

Murphy, B.R.; Chanock, R.M.: Genetic approaches to the prevention of influenza A virus infection; in Nayak, Genetic variation among influenza viruses. ICN-UCLA Symp., vol. 21, pp. 601–615 (Academic Press, New York 1981).

Murphy, B.R.; Sly, D.L.; Tierney, E.L.; Hosier, N.T.; Massicot, J.G.; London, W.T.; Chanock, R.M.; Webster, R.G.; Hinshaw, V.S.: Reassortant virus derived from avian and human influenza A virus is attenuated and immunogenic in monkeys. Science *218:* 1330 (1982).

Murphy, B.R.; Tolpin, M.D.; Massicot, J.; Kim, H.W.; Parrott, R.H.; Chanock, R.M.: Escape of a highly defective influenza A virus mutant from its *ts* phenotype by extragenic suppression and other types of mutation. Ann. N.Y. Acad. Sci. *354:* 142 (1980).

Nagata, S.; Taira, H.; Hall, A.; Johnsrud, L.; Steuli, M.; Escördi, J.; Boll, W.; Cantell, K.; Weissmann, C.: Synthesis in *E. coli* of a polypeptide with human leukocyte interferon activity. Nature, Lond. *284:* 316 (1980).

Nakano, J.H.; Hatch, M.H.; Thime, M.L.; Nottay, B.: Parameters for differentiating vaccine-derived and wild poliovirus strains. Prog. med. Virol., vol. 24, p. 178 (Karger, Basel 1978).

Nathanson, N.; Martin, J.R.: The epidemiology of poliomyelitis: enigmas surrounding its appearance, epidemicity, and disappearance. Am. J. Epidem. *110:* 672 (1979).

Naylor, P.T.; Larsen, H.S.; Huang, L.; Rouse, B.T.: In vivo induction of anti-herpes simplex virus immune response by type 1 antigens and lipid A incorporated into liposomes. Infect. Immunity *36:* 1209 (1982).

Naylor, S.L.; Sakaguchi, A.Y.; Shows, T.B.; Law, M.L.; Goeddel, D.V.; Gray, P.W.: Human immune interferon gene is located on chromosome 12. J. exp. Med. *157:* 1020 (1983).

Neff, B.J.; Weibel, R.E.; Buynak, E.B.; McLean, A.A.; Hilleman, M.R.: Clinical and laboratory studies of live cytomegalovirus vaccine Ad-169(40382). Proc. Soc. exp. Biol. Med. *160:* 32 (1979).

Neff, B.J.; Weibel, R.E.; Villarejos, V.M.; Buynak, E.B.; McLean, A.A.; Morton, D.H.; Wolanski, B.S.; Hilleman, M.R.: Clinical and laboratory studies of KMcC strain of live attenuated varicella virus (41071). Proc. Soc. exp. Biol. Med. *166:* 339 (1981).

Nightingale, E.O.: Recommendations for a national policy on poliomyelitis vaccination. New Engl. J. Med. *297:* 249 (1977).

Nilsen, A.E.; Aasen, T.; Halsos, A.M.; Kinge, B.R.; Tjotta, E.A.L.; Wikström, K.; Fiddian, A.P.: Efficacy of oral acyclovir in the treatment of initial and recurrent genital herpes. Lancet *ii:* 571 (1982).

Nilsen, T.W.; Baglioni, C.: A mechanism for discrimination between viral and host mRNA in interferon-treated cells. Proc. natn. Acad. Sci. USA *76:* 2600 (1979).

Nomoto, A.; Omata, T.; Toyoda, H.; Kuge, S.; Horie, H.; Kataoka, Y.; Genba, Y.; Nakano, Y.; Imura, N.: Complete nucleotide sequence of the attenuated poliovirus Sabin 1 strain genome. Proc. natn. Acad. Sci. USA *79:* 5793 (1982).

Norrby, E.: The effect of a carbobenzoxy tripeptide on the biological activities of measles virus. Virology *44:* 599 (1971).

North, J.R.; Morgan, A.J.; Thompson, J.L.; Epstein, M.A.: Purified EB virus gp 340 induces potent virus-neutralizing antibodies when incorporated in liposomes. Proc. natn. Acad. Sci. USA *79:* 7504 (1982).

North, T.W.; Cohen, S.S.: Aranucleosides and aranucleotides in viral chemotherapy. Pharmacol. Ther. *4:* 81 (1979).

Osborn, J.E.: Viral vaccines under development: a third generation. Adv. exp. Biol. med. Biol. *118:* 61 (1979).

Osborn, J.E.: Cytomegalovirus: pathogenicity, immunology, and vaccine initiatives. J. infect. Dis. *143:* 618 (1981).

Owerbach, D.; Rutter, W.J.; Shows, T.B.; Gray, P.; Goeddel, D.V.; Lawn, R.M.: Leukocyte and fibroblast interferon genes are located on human chromosome 9. Proc. natn. Acad. Sci. USA *78:* 3123 (1981).

Oxford, J.S. (ed.): Chemoprophylaxis and virus infections of the respiratory tract, vol. I, II (CRC Press, Cleveland 1977).

Oxford, J.S.; Galbraith, A.: Antiviral activity of amantadine: a review of laboratory and clinical data. Pharmacol. Ther. *11:* 181 (1980).

Palese, P.; Roizman, B. (eds.): Genetic variation of viruses. Ann. N.Y. Acad. Sci. *354:* (1980).

Pancic, F.; Steinberg, B.A.; Diana, G.D.; Carabateas, P.M.; Gorman, W.G.; Came, P.E.: Antiviral activity of WIN 41258-3, pyrazole compound, against herpes simplex virus in mouse genital infection and in guinea pig skin infection. Antimicrob. Agents Chemother. *19:* 470 (1981).

Panem, S.; Check, I.J.; Henriksen, D.; Vilček, J.: Alpha interferon and antibody to alpha interferon in systemic lupus erythematosus; in Merigan, Friedman, Interferons, UCLA Symp. on Mol. Cell. Biology, vol. XXV, pp. 233–240 (Academic Press, New York 1982).

Panicali, D.; Davis, S.W.; Weinberg, R.L.; Paoletti, E.: Construction of live vaccines by using genetically engineered poxviruses: biological activity of recombinant vaccinia virus expressing influenza virus hemagglutinin. Proc. natn. Acad. Sci. USA *80:* 5364 (1983).

Parks, W.P.; Rapp, F.: Prospects for herpesvirus vaccination – safety and efficacy considerations. Prog. med. Virol., vol. 21, p. 188 (Karger, Basel 1975).

Pavan-Langston, D.; Buchanan, R.A.; Alford, C.A.: Adenine arabinoside: an antiviral agent (North-Holland, Amsterdam 1975).

Pazin, G.J.; Ho, M.; Haverkos, H.W.; Armstrong, J.A.; Breinig, M.C.; Wechsler, H.L.; Arvin, A.M.; Merigan, T.C.; Cantell, K.: Effects of interferon-alpha on human warts. J. Interferon Res. *2:* 235 (1982).

Perkins, F.T.; Regamey, R.H. (eds.): Int. Symp. on influenza immunization. Dev. biol. Standard., vol. 39 (Karger, Basel 1977).

Pestka, S. (ed.): Interferons, parts A, B. Meth. Enzym. *78, 79* (1981).

Pestka, S.: The human interferons – from protein purification and sequence to cloning and expression in bacteria: before, between, and beyond. Archs Biochem. Biophys. *221:* 1 (1983).

Pestka, S.; Evinger, M.; Maeda, S.; Rehberg, E.; Familletti, P.C.; Kelder, B.: Biological properties of natural and recombinant interferons. Tex. Rep. Biol. Med. *41:* 31 (1982).

Pestka, S.; Maeda, S.; Hobbs, D.S.; Levy, W.P.; McCandliss, R.; Stein, S.; Moschera, J.A.; Staehelin, T.: The human interferons; in Mozes, Cellular responses to molecular modulators, pp. 455–493 (Academic Press, New York 1981).

Peterslund, N.A.; Seyer-Hansen, K.; Ipsen, J.; Esmann, V.; Schonheyder, H.; Juhl, H.: Acyclovir in herpes zoster. Lancet *ii:* 827 (1981).

Petricciani, J.C.; Hopps, H.E.; Chapple, P.J. (eds.): Cell substrates: their use in the production of vaccines and other biologicals. Adv. exp. med. Biol. *118* (Plenum Press, New York 1979).

Pfeffer, L.M.; Wang, E. Tamm, I.: Interferon effects on microfilament organization, cellular fibronectin distribution, and cell motility in human fibroblasts. J. Cell Biol. *85:* 9 (1980).

Phillpotts, R.J.; Jones, R.W.; Delong, D.C.; Reed, S.E.; Wallace, J.; Tyrrell, D.A.J.: The activity of enviroxime against rhinovirus infection in man. Lancet *i:* 1342 (1981).

Phillpotts, R.J.; Wallace, J.; Tyrrell, D.A.J.; Freestone, D.S.; Shepherd, W.M.: Failure of oral 4′,6-dichloroflavan to protect against rhinovirus infection in man. Archs Virol. *75:* 115 (1983).

Pitha, P.M.; Rowe, W.P.; Oxman, M.N.: Effect of interferon on exogenous, endogenous, and chronic murine leukemia virus infection. Virology *70:* 324 (1976).

Plotch, S.J.; Bouloy, M.; Krug, R.M.: Transfer of 5′-terminal cap of globin mRNA to influenza viral complementary RNA during transcription in vitro. Proc. natn. Acad. Sci. USA *76:* 1618 (1979).

Plotkin, S.A.: Rabies vaccine prepared in human cell cultures: progress and perspectives. Rev. infect. Dis. *2:* 433 (1980).

Pollard, R.B.: Interferons and interferon inducers: development of clinical usefulness and therapeutic promise. Drugs *23:* 37 (1982).

Pollard, R.B.; Egbert, P.R.; Gallagher, J.G.; Merigan, T.C.: Cytomegalovirus retinitis in immunosuppressed patients. I. Natural history and effects of treatment with adenine arabinoside. Ann. intern. Med. *93:* 655 (1980).

Pollard, R.B.; Merigan, T.C.: Experience with clinical applications of interferon and interferon inducers. Pharmacol. Ther. A *2:* 783 (1978).

Potter, C.W.: Inactivated influenza virus vaccine; in Beare, Basic and applied influenza research, chapt. 6 (CRC Press, Cleveland 1982).

Pourcel, C.; Sobzack, E.; Dubois, M.-F.; Gervais, M.; Drovet, J.; Tiollais, P.: Antigenicity and immunogenicity of hepatitis B virus particles produced by mouse cells transfected with cloned viral DNA. Virology *121:* 175 (1982).

Powers, C. N.; Peary, D. L.; Knight, V.: Selective inhibition of functional lymphocyte subpopulations by ribavirin. Antimicrob. Agents Chemother. *22:* 108 (1982).

Preble, O. T.; Black, R. J.; Klippel, J. H.; Friedman, R.; Vilček, J.: Interferon in systemic lupus erythematosus; in Merigan, Friedman, Interferons, UCLA Symp. on Mol. Cell. Biology, vol. XXV, pp. 219–231 (Academic Press, New York 1982).

Preblud, S. R.; Serdula, M. K.; Frank, J. A.; Brandling-Bennett, A. D.; Hinman, A. R.: Rubella vaccination in the United States: a ten-year review. Epidemiol. Rev. *2:* 171 (1980).

Preblud, S. R.; Stetler, H. C.; Frank, J. A.; Greaves, W. L.; Hinman, A. R.; Herrmann, K. L.: Fetal risk associated with rubella vaccine. J. Am. med. Ass. *246:* 1413 (1981).

Prince, A. M.; Ikram, H.; Hopp, T. P.: Hepatitis B virus vaccine: identification of HB_sAg/a and HB_sAg/d but not HB_sAg/y subtype antigenic determinants on a synthetic immunogenic peptide. Proc. natn. Acad. Sci. USA *79:* 579 (1982).

Provost, P. J.; Banker, F. S.; Giesa, P. A.; McAleer, W. J.; Buynak, E. B.; Hilleman, M. R.: Progress towards a live, attenuated human hepatitis A vaccine (41387). Proc. Soc. exp. Biol. Med. *170:* 8 (1982).

Provost, P. J.; Giesa, P. A.; McAleer, W. J.; Hilleman, M. R.: Isolation of hepatitis A virus in vitro in cell culture directly from human specimens. Proc. Soc. exp. Biol. Med. *167:* 201 (1981).

Provost, P. J.; Hilleman, M. R.: An inactivated hepatitis A virus vaccine prepared from infected marmoset liver. Proc. Soc. exp. Biol. Med. *159:* 201 (1978).

Purcell, R. H.; Gerin, J. L.: Hepatitis B vaccines: a status report; in Vyas, Cohen, Schmid, Viral hepatitis, p. 491 (Franklin Institute Press, Philadelphia 1978).

Purchase, H. G.: Prevention of Marek's disease: a review. Cancer Res. *36:* 696 (1976).

Racaniello, V. R.; Baltimore, D.: Cloned poliovirus complementary DNA is infectious in mammalian cells. Science *214:* 916 (1981).

Reid, L. M.; Minato, N.; Gresser, I.; Holland, J.; Kadish, A.; Bloom, B. R.: Influence of anti-mouse interferon serum on the growth and metastasis of tumor cells persistently infected with virus and of human prostatic tumors in athymic nude mice. Proc. natn. Acad. Sci. USA *78:* 1171 (1981).

Revel, M.: Molecular mechanisms involved in the antiviral effects of interferon; in Gresser, Interferon 1, pp. 102–163 (Academic Press, New York 1979).

Richardson, C. D.; Scheid, A.; Choppin, P. W.: Specific inhibition of paramyxovirus and myxovirus replication by oligopeptides with amino acid sequences similar to those at the N-termini of the F_1 or HA_2 viral polypeptides. Virology *105:* 205 (1980).

Richman, D. D.; Murphy, B. R.: The association of the temperature-sensitive phenotype with viral attenuation in animals and humans: implications for the development and use of live virus vaccines. Rev. infect. Dis. *1:* 413 (1979).

Richman, D. D.; Oxman, M. N.: Antiviral agents; in Weinstein, Fields, Seminars in infectious diseases, pp. 200–255 (Stratton Intercontinental, New York 1978).

Robbins, K. B.; Brandling-Bennett, A. D.; Hinman, A. R.: Low measles incidence: association with enforcement of school immunization laws. Am. J. publ. Hlth *71:* 270 (1981).

Roberts, W. K.; Hovanessian, A.; Brown, R. E.; Clemens, M. J.; Kerr, I. M.: Interferon-mediated protein kinase and low molecular weight inhibitor of protein synthesis. Nature, Lond. *264:* 477 (1976).

Roizman, B.; Warren, J.; Thuning, C. A.; Fanshaw, M. S.; Norrild, B.; Meignier, B.: Application of molecular genetics to the design of live herpes simplex virus vaccines. Dev. biol. Standard., vol. 52, pp. 287–304 (Karger, Basel 1982).

Romano, A.; Revel, M.; Guarari-Rotman, D.; Blumenthal, M.; Stein, R.: Use of human fibroblast-derived (beta) interferon in the treatment of epidemic adenovirus keratoconjunctivitis. J. Interferon Res. *1:* 95 (1980).

Rubin, B. Y.; Gupta, S. L.: Differential efficacies of human type I and type II interferons as antiviral and antiproliferative agents. Proc. natn. Acad. Sci. USA *77:* 5928 (1980).

Rubinstein, M.; Levy, W. P.; Moschera, J. A.; Lai, C.-Y.; Hershberg, R. D.; Bartlett, R. T.; Pestka, S.: Human leukocyte interferon: isolation and characterization of several molecular forms. Archs Biochem. Biophys. *210:* 307 (1981).

Rubinstein, M.; Rubinstein, S.; Familletti, P. C.; Miller, R. S.; Waldman, A. A.; Pestka, S.: Human leukocyte interferon: production, purification to homogeneity and initial characterization. Proc. natn. Acad. Sci. USA *76:* 640 (1979).

Sabin, A. B.: Amantadine and influenza: evaluation of conflicting reports. J. infect. Dis. *138:* 557 (1978).

Sabin, A. B.: Vaccination against poliomyelitis in economically underdeveloped countries. Bull. Wld Hlth Org. *58:* 141 (1980).

Sabin, A. B.: Immunization: evaluation of some currently available and prospective vaccines. J. Am. med. Ass. *246:* 236 (1981a).

Sabin, A. B.: Paralytic poliomyelitis: old dogmas and new perspectives. Rev. infect. Dis. *3:* 543 (1981b).

Sabin, A. B.; Arechiga, A. F.; de Castro, J. F.; Sever, J. L.; Madden, D. L.; Shekarchi, I.; Albrecht, P.: Successful immunization of children with and without maternal antibody by aerosolized measles vaccine. J. Amer. med. Assoc. *249:* 2651 (1983).

Sagar, A. D.; Pickering, L. A.; Sussman-Berger, P.; Stewart, W. E.; Sehgal, P. B.: Heterogeneity of interferon mRNA species from Sendai virus-induced human lymphoblastoid (Namalva) cells and Newcastle disease virus-induced murine fibroblastoid (L) cells. Nucl. Acids Res. *9:* 149 (1981).

Sagar, A. D.; Sehgal, P. B.; Slate, D. L.; Ruddle, F. H.: Multiple human β interferon genes. J. exp. Med. *156:* 744 (1982).

Salk, D.: Eradication of poliomyelitis in the United States. I, II, III. Rev. infect. Dis. *2:* 228–273 (1980).

Salk, J.; Salk, D.: Control of influenza and poliomyelitis with killed virus vaccines. Science *195:* 834 (1977).

Sanchez, Y.; Ionescu-Matiu, I.; Dreesman, G. R.; Kramp, W.; Six, H. R.; Hollinger, F. B.; Melnick, J. L.: Humoral and cellular immunity to hepatitis B virus-derived antigens: comparative activity of Freund complete adjuvant, alum and liposomes. Infect. Immunity *30:* 728 (1980).

Saral, R.; Burns, W. H.; Laskin, O. L.; Santos, G. W.; Lietman, P. S.: Acyclovir prophylaxis of herpes-simplex-virus infections: a randomized, double-blind, controlled trial in bone-marrow-transplant recipients. New Engl. J. Med. *305:* 63 (1981).

Schaeffer, H. J.; Beauchamp, L.; deMiranda, P.; Elion, G. B.; Bauer, D. J.; Collins, P.: 9-(2-Hydroxyethoxymethyl) guanine activity against viruses of the herpes group. Nature, Lond. *272:* 583 (1978).

Schmidt, A.; Chernajovsky, Y.; Shulman, L.; Federman, P.; Berissi, H.; Revel, M.: An interferon-induced phosphodiesterase degrading (2′-5′)oligoisoadenylate and the C-C-A terminus of tRNA. Proc. natn. Acad. Sci. USA *76:* 4788 (1979).

Schnipper, L. E.; Crumpacker, C. S.: Resistance of herpes simplex virus to acycloguanosine: role of viral thymidine kinase and DNA polymerase loci. Proc. natn. Acad. Sci. USA *77:* 2270 (1980).

Scholtissek, C.; Faulkner, G. P.: Amantadine resistant and sensitive influenza A strains and recombinants. J. gen. Virol. *44:* 807 (1979).

Schonberger, L. B.; Bregman, D. J.; Sullivan-Bolyai, J. Z.; Keenlyside, R. A.; Ziegler, D. W.; Retailliau, H. F.; Eddins, D. L.; Bryan, J. A.: Guillain-Barré syndrome following vaccination in the National Influenza Immunization Program, United States, 1976–1977. Am. J. Epidem. *110:* 105 (1979).

Schultz, R. M.; Papamatheakis, J. D.; Chirigos, M. A.: Interferon: an inducer of macrophage activation by polyanions. Science *197:* 674 (1977).

Scott, G. J.; Secher, D. S.; Flowers, D.; Bate, J.; Cantell, K.; Tyrrell, D. A. J.: The clinical toxicity of interferon. Br. med. J. *282:* 1345 (1981).

Scott, G. M.; Phillpotts, R. J.; Wallace, J.; Gauci, C. L.; Greiner, J.; Tyrrell, D. A. J.: Prevention of rhinovirus colds by human interferon alpha-2 from *Escherichia coli.* Lancet *ii:* 186 (1982).

Scott, G. M.; Tyrrell, D. A. J.: Interferon: therapeutic fact or fiction for the 1980s? Br. med. J. *280:* 1558 (1980).

Scullard, G. H.; Pollard, R. B.; Smith, J. L.; Sacks, S. L.; Gregory, P. B.; Robinson, W. S.; Merigan, T. C.: Antiviral treatment of chronic hepatitis B virus infection. I. Changes in viral markers with interferon combined with adenine arabinoside. J. infect. Dis. *143:* 772 (1981).

Secher, D. S.: Immunoradiometric assay of human leukocyte interferon using monoclonal antibody. Nature, Lond. *290:* 501 (1981).

Secher, D. S.; Burke, D. C.: A monoclonal antibody for large-scale purification of human leukocyte interferon. Nature, Lond. *285:* 446 (1980).

Sehgal, P. B.; Sagar, A. D.; Braude, I. A.: Further heterogeneity of human α interferon mRNA species. Science *214:* 803 (1981).

Sela, M.; Arnon, R.: Antiviral antibodies obtained with aqueous solution of a synthetic antigen; in Mizrahi et al., New developments with human and veterinary vaccines. Prog. clin. biol. Res. *47:* 315 (Liss, New York 1980).

Selby, P. J.; Powles, R. L.; Jameson, B.; Kay, H. E. M.; Watson, J. G.; Thornton, R.; Morgenstern, G.; Clink, H. M.; McElwain, T. J.; Prentice, H. G.; Corringham, R.; Ross, M. G.; Hoffbrand, A. V.; Brigden, D.: Parenteral acyclovir therapy for herpesvirus infections in man. Lancet *ii:* 1267 (1979).

Sen, G. C.; Shaila, S.; Lebleu, B.; Brown, G. E.; Desrosierd, R. C.; Lengyel, P.: Impairment of reovirus mRNA methylation in extracts of interferon-treated Ehrlich ascites tumor cells: further characteristics of the phenomenon. J. Virol. *21:* 69 (1977).

Shannon, W.; Schabel, F.: Antiviral agents as adjuncts in cancer chemotherapy. Pharmacol. Ther. *11:* 263 (1980).

Sidwell, R. W.; Robins, R. K.; Hillyard, I. W.: Ribavirin: an antiviral agent. Pharmacol. Ther. *6:* 123 (1979).

Simons, K.; Helenius, A.; Leonard, K.; Sarvas, M.; Gething, M. J.: Formation of protein micelles from amphiphilic membrane proteins. Proc. natn. Acad. Sci. USA *75:* 5306 (1978).

Simons, K.; Helenius, A.; Morein, B.; Balcorova, J.; Sharp, M.: Development of effective subunit vaccines against enveloped viruses; in Mizrahi, New developments with human and veterinary vaccines. Prog. clin. biol. Res. *47:* 217 (Liss, New York 1980).

Skehel, J. J.; Hay, A. J.; Armstrong, J. A.: On the mechanism of inhibition of influenza virus replication by amantadine hydrochloride. J. gen. Virol. *38:* 97 (1978).

Skelly, J.; Howard, C. R.; Zuckerman, A. J.: Hepatitis B polypeptide vaccine preparation in micelle form. Nature, Lond. *290:* 51 (1981).

Smith, G. L.; Mackett, M.; Moss, B.: Infectious vaccinia virus recombinants that express hepatitis B surface antigen. Nature, Lond. *302:* 490 (1983).

Smith, K. O.; Galloway, K. S.; Kennell, W. L.; Ogilvie, K. K.; Radatus, B. K.: A new nucleoside analog, 9-[[2-hydroxy-1-(hydroxymethyl) ethoxy] methyl]guanine, highly active in vitro against herpes simplex virus types 1 and 2. Antimicrob. Agents Chemother. *22:* 55 (1982).

Smith, R. A.; Kirkpatrick, W. (eds.): Ribavirin – a broad spectrum antiviral agent (Academic Press, New York 1980).

Smith, R. A.; Sidwell, R. W.; Robins, R. K.: Antiviral mechanisms of action. A. Rev. Pharmacol. Toxicol. *20:* 259 (1980).

Sonnenfeld, G.; Mandel, A. D.; Merigan, T. C.: Time and dosage dependence of immunoenhancement by murine type II interferon preparations. Cell. Immunol. *40:* 285 (1978).

Sonnenfeld, G.; Merigan, T. C.: The role of interferon in viral infections. Springer Semin. Immunopathol. *2:* 311 (1979).

Spruance, S. L.; Schnipper, L. E.; Overall, J. C.; Kern, E. R.; Webster, B.; Modlin, J.; Wenerstrom, G.; Burton, C.; Arndt, K. A.; Chiu, G. L.; Crumpacker, C. S.: Treatment of herpes simplex labialis with topical acyclovir in polyethylene glycol. J. infect. Dis. *146:* 85 (1982).

Staehelin, T.; Hobbs, D. S.; Kung, H.-F.; Lai, C.-Y.; Pestka, S.: Purification and characterization of recombinant human leukocyte interferon (IFLrA) with monoclonal antibodies. J. biol. Chem. *256:* 9750 (1981a).

Staehelin, T.; Stähli, C.; Hobbs, D. S.; Pestka, S.: A rapid quantitative assay of high sensitivity for human leukocyte interferon with monoclonal antibodies. Meth. Enzym. *79:* 589 (1981b).

Starr, S. E.; Glazer, J. P.; Friedman, H. M.; Farquhar, J. D.; Plotkin, S. A.: Specific cellular and humoral immunity after immunization with live Towne strain cytomegalovirus vaccine. J. infect. Dis. *143:* 585 (1981).

Sternberg, M. J. E.; Cohen, F. E.: Prediction of the secondary and tertiary structures of interferon from four homologous amino acid sequences. Int. J. biol. Macromol. *4:* 137 (1982).

Stewart, W. E.: The interferon system (Springer, Vienna 1979).

Stewart, W. E.; de Clercq, E.; Billiau, A.; Desmyter, J.; de Somer, P.: Increased susceptibility of cells treated with interferon to the toxicity of polyriboinosinic acid polyribocytidylic acid. Proc. natn. Acad. Sci. USA *69:* 1851 (1972).

Stiehm, E. R.: Interferon: immunobiology and clinical significance. Annals, int. Med. *96:* 80 (1982).

Stokes, J.; Weibel, R.E.; Villarejos, V.M.; Arguedas, J.A.; Buynak, E.B.; Hilleman, M.R.: Trivalent combined measles-mumps-rubella vaccine. J. Am. med. Ass. *218:* 57 (1971).

Strander, H.: Anti-tumor effects of interferons and its possible use as an anti-neoplastic agent in man. Tex. Rep. Biol. Med. *35:* 429 (1977).

Straus, S.; Seidlin, M.; Takiff, H.; Bachrach, S.; DiGiovanna, J.; Western, K.; Creagh-Kirk, T.; Lininger, L.; Alling, D.: Suppression of recurrent genital herpes with oral acyclovir. Clin. Res. *31/2:* 543A (1983).

Streuli, M.; Hall, A.; Boll, W.; Stewart, W.E.; Nagata, S.; Weissmann, C.: Target cell specificity of two species of human interferon-α produced in *Escherichia coli* and of hybrid molecules derived from them. Proc. natn. Acad. Sci. USA *78:* 2848 (1981).

Stridh, S.; Oberg, B.; Chattopadhyaya, J.; Josephson, S.: Functional analysis of influenza RNA polymerase activity by the use of caps, oligonucleotides and polynucleotides. Antiviral Res. *1:* 97 (1981).

Stringfellow, D.A.: Interferon and interferon inducers (Dekker, New York 1980a).

Stringfellow, D.A.: Interferon inducers: theory and experimental application; in Stringfellow, Interferon and interferon inducers, pp. 145–165 (Dekker, New York 1980b).

Sundmacher, R.: Interferon in ocular viral diseases; in Gresser, Interferon 4 (Academic Press, London 1982).

Sveda, M.M.; Lai, C.-J.: Functional expression in primate cells of cloned DNA coding for the hemagglutinin surface glycoprotein of influenza virus. Proc. natn. Acad. Sci. USA *78:* 5488 (1981).

Sveda, M.M.; Markoff, L.J.; Lai, C.-J.: Cell surface expression of the influenza virus hemagglutinin requires the hydrophobic carboxy-terminal sequences. Cell *30:* 649 (1982).

Swallow, D.L.: Antiviral agents. Prog. Drug Res. *22:* 267 (1978).

Szmuness, W.; Alter, H.J.; Maynard, J.M. (eds.): Viral hepatitis (Franklin Institute Press, Philadelphia 1982).

Szmuness, W.; Stevens, C.E.; Harley, E.J.; Zang, E.A.; Oleszko, W.R.; William, D.C.; Sadovsky, R.; Morrison, J.M.; Kellner, A.: Hepatitis B vaccine: demonstration of efficacy in a controlled clinical trial in a high-risk population in the United States. New Engl. J. Med. *303:* 833 (1980).

Szmuness, W.; Stevens, C.E.; Harley, E.J.; Zang, E.A.; Taylor, P.E.; Alter, H.J.; the Dialysis Vaccine Trial Group: The immune response of healthy adults to a reduced dose of hepatitis B vaccine. J. med. Virol. *8:* 123 (1981a).

Szmuness, W.; Stevens, C.E.; Oleszko, W.R.; Goodman, A.: Passive-active immunization against hepatitis B: immunogenicity studies in adult Americans. Lancet *i:* 575 (1981b).

Takahashi, M.; Asano, Y.; Kamiya, H.; Baba, K.; Yamanishi, K.: Active immunization for varicella-zoster virus; in Nahmias, Dowdle, Schinazi, The human herpesviruses, pp. 414–431 (Elsevier, New York 1981).

Taniguchi, T.; Guarente, L.; Roberts, T.M.; Kimelman, D.; Douhan, J.; Ptashne, M.: Expression of the human fibroblast interferon gene in *Escherichia coli.* Proc. natn. Acad. Sci. USA *77:* 5230 (1980a).

Taniguchi, T.; Mantei, N.; Schwarzstein, M.; Nagata, S.; Muramatsu, M.; Weissmann, C.: Human leukocyte and fibroblast interferons are structurally related. Nature, Lond. *285:* 547 (1980b).

Taylor, J. L.; Grossberg, S. E.: Chemical induction of interferon: carboxymethylacridanone and other low molecular weight chemicals. Tex. Rep. Biol. Med. *41:* 158 (1982).

Taylor-Papadimitriou, J.: Effects of interferons on cell growth and function; in Gresser, Interferon 2, pp. 13–46 (Academic Press, New York 1980).

Tenser, R. B.; Miller, R. L.; Rapp, F.: Trigeminal ganglion infection by thymidine kinase-negative mutants of herpes simplex virus. Science *205:* 915 (1979).

Tidwell, R. R.; Geratz, J. D.; Dann, O.; Volz, G.; Zeh, D.; Loewe, H.: Diarylamidine derivatives with one or both of the aryl moieties consisting of an indole or indole-like ring. Inhibitors of arginine-specific esteroproteases. J. medicinal Chem. *21:* 613 (1978).

Tisdale, M.; Selway, J. W. T.: Inhibition of an early stage of rhinovirus replication by dichloroflavan (BW683C). J. gen. Virol. *64:* 795 (1983).

Torrence, P. F.; de Clercq, E.: Inducers and induction of interferons. Pharmacol. Ther. A *2:* 1 (1977).

Trinchieri, G.; Santoli, D.: Antiviral activity induced by culturing lymphocytes with tumor-derived or virus-transformed cells. Enhancement of human natural killer cell activity by interferon and antagonistic inhibition of susceptibility of target cells to lysis. J. exp. Med. *147:* 1314 (1978).

Tyeryar, F. J.; Richardson, L. S.; Belshe, R. B.: Report of a workshop on respiratory syncytial virus and parainfluenza viruses. J. infect. Dis. *137:* 835 (1978).

Tyrrell, D. A. J.; Schild, G. C.; Dowdle, W. R.; Chanock, R. M.; Murphy, B. R.: Development and use of influenza vaccines. Bull. Wld Hlth Org. *59:* 165 (1981).

Tyrrell, D. A. J.; Smith, J. W. G.: Vaccination against influenza A. Br. med. Bull. *35:* 77 (1979).

Valenzuela, P.; Medina, A.; Rutter, W. J.; Ammerer, G.; Hall, B. D.: Synthesis and assembly of hepatitis B virus surface antigen particles in yeast. Nature, Lond. *298:* 347 (1982).

van Damme, J.; Billiau, A.: Large scale production of human fibroblast interferon. Meth. Enzym. *78:* 101 (1981).

van Wezel, A. L.: Present state and developments in the production of inactivated poliomyelitis vaccine. Dev. biol. Standard., vol. 47, p. 7 (Karger, Basel 1981).

van Wezel, A. L.; van Steenis, G.; Hannik, C. A.; Cohen, H.: New approach to the production of concentrated and purified inactivated polio and rabies tissue culture vaccines. Dev. biol. Standard., vol. 41, p. 159 (Karger, Basel 1978).

Vilček, J.; Gresser, I.; Merigan, T. C. (eds.): Regulatory functions of interferons. Ann. N.Y. Acad. Sci. *350:* 1–641 (1980).

Vilček, J.; Havell, E. A.; Yamazaki, S.: Superinduction of interferon with metabolic inhibitors: possible mechanisms and practical applications. J. infect. Dis. *133:* A22 (1976).

Vilček, J.; Yip, Y. K.; Pang, R. H. L.; Thayer, K.; Henriksen, D.; Zerebeckyj-Eckhardt, I.; Urban, C.; Taniguchi, T.: How many interferons are there? in Mozes, Cellular responses to molecular modulators, pp. 331–345 (Academic Press, New York 1981).

Virelizier, J.-L.; Gresser, I.: Role of interferon in the pathogenesis of viral diseases of mice as demonstrated by the use of anti-interferon serum. V. Protective role in mouse hepatitis virus type 3 infection of susceptible and resistant strains of mice. J. Immun. *120:* 1616 (1978).

Vyas, G.; Cohen, S. N.; Schmid, R. (eds.): Viral hepatitis (Franklin Institute press, Philadelphia 1978).

Walker, R. T.; de Clercq, E.; Eckstein, F.: Nucleoside analogues (Plenum Press, New York 1979).

Wallin, J.; Lernestedt, J.O.; Lycke, E.; Ogenstad, S.: Topical treatment of recurrent genital herpes infection with foscarnet. Abstr. 5th Int. Meet. Int. Soc. Sexually Transmitted Disease Research, p. 181 (1983).

Walsh, J.A.; Warren, K.S.: Selective primary health care. An interim strategy for disease control in developing countries. New Engl. J. Med. *301:* 967 (1979).

Watanabe, K.A.; Reichman, U.; Hirota, K.; Lopez, C.; Fox, J.J.: Nucleosides. 110. Synthesis and antiherpes virus activity of some 2′-fluoro-2′-deoxyarabinofuranosylpyrimidine nucleosides. J. medicinal Chem. *22:* 21 (1979).

Watson, R.J.; Weis, J.H.; Salstrom, J.S.; Enquist, L.W.: Herpes simplex type-1 glycoprotein D gene: nucleotide sequence and expression in *Escherichia coli.* Science *218:* 381 (1982).

Webster, R.G.; Laver, W.G.; Air, G.M.; Schild, G.C.: Molecular mechanisms of variation in influenza viruses. Nature, Lond. *296:* 115 (1982).

Weibel, R.E.; Buynak, E.B.; McLean, A.A.; Hilleman, M.R.: Follow-up surveillance for antibody in human subjects following live attenuated measles, mumps and rubella virus vaccines. Proc. Soc. exp. Biol. Med. *162:* 328 (1979).

Weil, J.; Epstein, C. J.; Epstein, L.B.; Sedmak, J. J.; Sabran, J.L.; Grossberg, S.E.: A unique set of polypeptides is induced by γ interferon in addition to those induced in common with α and β interferons. Nature, Lond. *301:* 437 (1983).

Weis, J.H.; Enquist, L.W.; Salstrom, J.S.; Watson, R.J.: An immunologically active chimaeric protein containing herpes simplex virus type 1 glycoprotein D. Nature, Lond. *302:* 72 (1983).

Weissenbach, J.; Chernajovsky, Y.; Zeevi, M.; Shulman, K.; Soreq, H.; Nir, U.; Wallach, D.; Perricaudet, M.; Tiollais, P.; Revel, M.: Two interferon mRNAs in human fibroblasts: in vitro translation and *Escherichia coli* cloning studies. Proc. natn. Acad. Sci. USA *77:* 7152 (1980).

Weissmann, C.: The cloning of interferon and other mistakes; in Gresser, Interferon 3, pp. 101–134 (Academic Press, New York 1981).

Weissmann, C.; Nagata, S.; Boll, W.; Fountoulakis, M.; Fujisawa, A.; Fujisawa, J.I.; Haynes, J.; Henco, K.; Mantei, N.; Ragg, H.; Schein, C.; Schmid, J.; Shaw, G.; Streuli, M.; Taira, H.; Todokoro, K.; Weidle, U.: Structure and expression of human alpha-interferon genes; in Merigan, Friedman, Interferons, UCLA Symp. on Mol. Cell. Biology, vol. XXV, pp. 295–326 (Academic Press, New York 1982).

Wellings, S.P.C.; Awdry, P.N.; Bors, F.H.; Jones, B.R.; Brown, D.C.; Kaufman, H.E.: Critical evaluation of trifluorothymidine in the treatment of herpes simplex corneal ulcers. Am. J. Ophthal. *73:* 932 (1972).

Wetzel, R.; Levine, H.L.; Estell, D.A.; Shire, S.; Finer-Moore, J.; Stroud, R.M.; Bewley, T.A.: Structure-function studies on human alpha interferon; in Merigan, Friedman, Interferons, UCLA Symp. on Mol. Cell. Biology, vol. XXV, pp. 365–376 (Academic Press, New York 1982).

Wheelock, E.F.: Interferon-like virus-inhibitor induced in human leukocytes by phytohemagglutinin. Science *149:* 310 (1965).

Whitley, R.J.; Alford, C.A.: Developmental aspects of selected antiviral chemotherapeutic agents. A. Rev. Microbiol. *32:* 285 (1978).

Whitley, R.J.; Alford, C.A.: Parenteral antiviral chemotherapy of human herpesviruses; in Nahmias, The human herpesviruses, pp. 478–489 (Elsevier, New York 1981).

Whitley, R.J.; Soong, S.-J.; Dolin, R.; Betts, R.; Linnemann, C.; Alford, C.A.; the NIAID

Collaborative Antiviral Study Group: Early vidarabine therapy to control the complications of herpes zoster in immunosuppressed patients. New Engl. J. Med. *307:* 971 (1982).

Whitley, R.J.; Soong, S.-J.; Hirsch, M.S.; Karchmer, A.W.; Dolin, R.; Galasso, G.; Dunnick, J.K.; Alford, C.A.; the NIAID Collaborative Antiviral Study Group: Herpes simplex encephalitis: vidarabine therapy and diagnostic problems. New Engl. J. Med. *304:* 313 (1981).

Wiktor, T.J.; Koprowski, H.: Does the existence of rabies antigenic variants warrant re-evaluation of rabies vaccines? in Proc. 1st Int. Conf. on The Impact of Viral Diseases on the Development of Latin American Countries and the Caribbean Region (1982).

Wiktor, T.J.; Plotkin, S.A.; Koprowski, H.: Development and clinical trials of the new human rabies vaccine of tissue culture (human diploid cell) origin. Dev. biol. Standard., vol. 40, p. 3 (Karger, Basel 1978).

Wiley, D.C.; Wilson, I.A.; Skehel, J.J.: Structural identification of the antibody binding sites of Hong Kong influenza haemagglutinin and their involvement in antigenic variation. Nature, Lond. *289:* 373 (1981).

Wilson, I.A.; Skehel, J.J.; Wiley, D.C.: Structure of the hemagglutinin membrane glycoprotein of influenza virus at 3 Å resolution. Nature, Lond. *289:* 366 (1981).

WHO Consultative Group: The relation between persisting spinal paralysis and poliomyelitis vaccine – results of a ten-year enquiry. Bull. Wld Hlth Org. *60:* 231 (1982).

World Health Organization: WHO Expert Committee on Yellow Fever, Third Report. Tech. Rep. Ser. Wld Hlth Org. *479* (WHO, Geneva 1971).

World Health Organization: Immunological adjuvants. Tech. Rep. Ser. Wld Hlth Org. *595* (WHO, Geneva 1976).

World Health Organization: Interferon therapy. Tech. Rep. Ser. Wld Hlth Org. *676* (WHO, Geneva 1982).

World Health Organization: Viral vaccines and antiviral drugs. Tech. Rep. Ser. Wld Hlth Org. 693 (WHO, Geneva 1983).

Wright, P.F.; Okabe, N.; McKee, K.T.; Maassab, H.F.; Karzon, D.T.: Cold-adapted recombinant influenza A virus vaccines in seronegative young children. J. infect. Dis. *146:* 71 (1982).

Wunner, W.H.; Dietzschold, B.; Curtis, P.J.; Wiktor, T.J.: Rabies subunit vaccines. J. gen. Virol. *64;* 1649 (1983).

Yatvin, M.B.; Weinstein, J.N.; Dennis, W.H.; Blumenthal, R.: Design of liposomes for enhanced local release of drugs by hyperthermia. Science *202:* 1290 (1978).

Yelverton, E.; Leung, D.; Weck, P.; Gray, P.W.; Goeddel, D.V.: Bacterial synthesis of a novel human leukocyte interferon. Nucl. Acids Res. *9:* 731 (1981).

Yelverton, E.; Norton, S.; Obijeski, J.F.; Goeddel, D.V.: Rabies virus glycoprotein analogs: biosynthesis in *Escherichia coli.* Science *219:* 614 (1983).

Yip, Y.K.; Barrowclough, B.; Urban, C.; Vilček, J.: Purification of two subspecies of human gamma (immune) interferon. Proc. natn. Acad. Sci. USA *79:* 1820 (1982).

Zamecnik, P.C.; Stephenson, M.L.: Inhibition of Rous sarcoma virus replication and cell transformation by a specific oligodeoxynucleotide. Proc. natn. Acad. Sci. USA *75:* 280 (1978).

Zoon, K.C.; Smith, M.E.; Brigden, P.J.; zur Nedden, D.; Anfinsen, C.B.: Purification and partial characterization of human lymphoblastoid interferon. Proc. natn. Acad. Sci. USA *76:* 5601 (1979).